THE DANCING HEALERS

A Doctor's Journey of Healing with Native Americans

Carl A. Hammerschlag, M.D.

1817

Harper & Row, Publishers, San Francisco

New York, Grand Rapids, Philadelphia, St. Louis
London, Singapore, Sydney, Tokyo, Toronto

FIRST HARPER & ROW PAPERBACK EDITION PUBLISHED IN 1989.

Library of Congress Cataloging-in-Publication Data

Hammerschlag, Carl A.
    The dancing healers : a doctor's journey of healing with native
    Americans / Carl A. Hammerschlag. — 1st ed.
        pg. cm.
    ISBN 0-06-250395-4
    ISBN 0-06-250395-2 (pbk.)
    1. Indians of North America—Southwest, New—Medicine.
    2. Hammerschlag, Carl A.   I. Title
    E78.S7H23   1988
615.8′51—dc19   87-45704

89 90 91 92 93 BANTA 10 9 8 7 6 5 4 3

CONTENTS

PREFACE

Milton Erickson, that master hypnotherapist, understood that to begin a story by saying "Remember when" was already to begin to place the audience into an altered state of consciousness—the very act of remembering is a kind of trance in itself. Erickson also knew that when you tell a story, you are speaking directly to the unconscious, the very essence of the listener.

My twenty years in Indian country have shown me the great, universal power inherent in the stories we have told each other in all cultures throughout all of time. There are heroes; there are monsters. People die; they are reborn. And there are miracles.

When we see this universal connection among all who have walked the earth, it becomes clear that all history is the history of our own time. All stories speak to each of us. Understanding this connection is crucial if we're to be able to live together and to live with ourselves. We must learn to feel how other people connect to one another and to the universe.

No one makes it alone. We must all be connected to something other than ourselves—to others on our walk and to something outside all of us. At the same time, in this everlasting now, each of us is unique. We each have our own truth and our own power, and that is what we must follow.

These are the stories I have lived. They tell of how I began to learn to become a healer rather than a doctor. They tell of how I came to understand that the power to heal comes from hearing your own music and dancing your own dance.

ACKNOWLEDGMENTS

It was the old Indian men who told me that I should tell the stories. It has not been easy. For eight years I have picked the manuscript up and put it down.

Would my motives be suspect? Would I be ridiculed? Would the visibility compromise my credibility?

Enough already. Listen to the stories. They are not mine. I just heard them.

They are all true. I have changed some names and places to protect the anonymity of those who chose to remain unnamed. The words are mine, in the best way I know how to write them. If the stories do not move you, it is because I could not write them as well as I learned them.

I have never seen or walked the path alone. The book is for my family, friends, teachers, patients, and students who have walked with me. It is with love for my wife and children who made the painful and enlightening journey near, if not always by, my side.

It is with thanks to Brad Steiger, Phyllis Steckler, Carol Sowell, Tom Grady, and Ann Moru, who felt my heart and showed me how to share it better. To Dennis Numkena, visionary artist, whose cover design illuminates the Hopi symbols of the healing dance.

And it is for these mentors, their light still shines;

Santiago Rosetta 1893–1975
Arno Hammerschlag 1905–1977
Herbert Talaheftewa 1903–1979
Bill Dalton 1897–1981

Erich Fromm 1900–1980
Milton Erickson 1901–1980
Brave Buffalo (Devere
   Eastman) 1930–1987

Mi takuye oyacin
To all my relations
C.A.H.

Introduction

SANTIAGO'S DANCE

In 1965, after I had completed my medical internship at the Public Health Service Hospital in Seattle, Washington, I entered the Indian Health Service. It made more sense to me than going to Vietnam, a real possibility for someone who was twenty-six years old in that year and a recent graduate from the Upstate Medical Center in Syracuse, New York. Serving with the IHS would fulfill my military obligation. And since no one knows more than someone who has just graduated from medical school, I went to the Indian country of the Southwest to help, to offer healing to the people.

Yet I was also a child. I was terrified of so many things. I had not yet learned that it is all right not to be always sure of everything.

I was a child of my time, an activist in support of the radical causes and beliefs of that day: end the war, help the underdog, listen to the uncorrupted people who live next to the earth. I wanted to work among people I had feelings for, the disenfranchised and the neglected.

Why I chose an Indian reservation in the Southwest rather than the ghettoes of the Eastern cities in which I had grown up was harder to say. The Southwest rang with a certain mystery; I had a romantic vision of a unique culture. I didn't know then why the Southwest drew me, but I had a sense there was something there to be learned.

And indeed, after more than twenty years among the native people of the Southwest, I now know that my further education, my unfinished business with my own history and my own demons, the things I needed to know to be able to help myself and others—those were the real reasons I came to this beautiful, mysterious country.

During my education at the City College of New York and the State University of New York Medical School, my plan was to be a "real doctor," a family practitioner. I would hang a shingle someplace and let people pay me in chickens and pigs. I thought I could bring healing to plain people who would gratefully welcome my expertness. I was ready to save the world—people needed me. Most of us go into medicine to try to "do it" for somebody.

I didn't know I was going to the Southwest to be healed myself.

The IHS sent me to Sante Fe, New Mexico, as a General Medical Officer assigned to the Pueblo tribes along the Rio Grande. The very name rang with magic! The Rio Grande. How exotic.

I came with a wife and two small daughters. Elaine and I had met when I was nineteen and a premedical student; she was a nurse. It was the familiar doctor-nurse pairing: young nurse marries young med student and helps put him through school. We survived the stresses of the process and managed to transform the struggle into a growing family.

I was a big-city boy from the concrete canyons of the East who thought you needed to be immunized against yellow fever if you were foolhardy enough to cross the George Washington Bridge. I knew nothing of the Pueblo tribes. I knew Indians only from Hollywood's shallow presentations. And in those sagas I had always cheered for the Indians against the cowboys, because of my sympathy for the apparent underdog in any situation.

But Santa Fe immediately began chipping away at my brand new M.D. bravado. It was the smallest town Elaine and I had ever seen, and I found that many of those I had come to help hated me simply because I was a white man. As a child of the Jewish nightmares of World War II, I could certainly identify with the Indians' terrible sense of disenfranchisement, but I could not relate to being hated simply for being white.

I worked in the Santa Fe Indian Hospital under direction of an old doc who had been there for many years. The hospital was a collection of huge wards. You could go from one bed to the next just by moving the "chart cart" six inches down.

The pace was killing. I worked seven days a week. Another young doctor and I were on call every other night and every other weekend. Lunch got eaten while I moved from one room to another. I had expected to work long and hard, but I didn't expect to be seeing one hundred people a day, to have no time to think and no energy for my family. It didn't take me long to realize I wasn't up to the rigors of a life as a general practitioner in that kind of setting.

The conditions we saw were distressing and we functioned in a constant state of emergency. Members of the Pueblo tribes came to us with every kind of ailment—gastric ulcers, tuberculosis, heart attacks, cancers. The rate of infant mortality was high and it wasn't unusual to see children with 5-to-10-percent dehydration, the result of severe diarrhea. These children were so shriveled we had to shave their scalps to find veins where we could inject the intravenous fluid needed to restore health.

Despite these conditions, the Pueblos were reluctant to come to the hospital to see doctors. For them an illness would either get better or it wouldn't and a hospital was a place you went to die.

What we saw as their passivity frustrated us. What we didn't know was that there was another system, another way of dealing with living and dying, suffering and healing, that we knew nothing of. We young smart docs thought we could do more than we really could and knew more than we did.

Since ours was the only medical service and we were the only doctors on the reservation, two days a week I went out into the villages. The Indian Health Service had only started in 1955. Before that, the Bureau of Indian Affairs (BIA) in the Department of the Interior ran such hospitals as there were. And during World War II, Indian facilities were last on the list to receive supplies and personnel. I was unprepared for the results of this long-time neglect.

I saw a rare liver disease in a previously healthy twenty-year-old woman who delivered a quite jaundiced, stillborn child and then died herself within twenty-four hours. It transpired so quickly that I felt I never knew what happened.

I had a patient whose heart valves were being nibbled away by bacteria that had invaded his blood after he had cut himself while skinning a rabbit. In spite of vigorous treatment, I watched him die from blood poisoning in six weeks.

I lost a thirty-year-old chronic alcoholic in delerium tremens. He drowned in his own secretions, an unlikely complication of that disease I had been taught.

There was dying all around me, for which I was not well prepared. It made me worry about my competence and my training. Some people afflicted with a disease got well, while others who suffered from the same malady died from it. Certain men and women who were exposed to a disease never got it at all.

Many of the women delivered their babies squatting on sheepskins so that the first thing the child would touch was the Earth, the mother of us all. They refused to get on the table and give birth on their backs. When they would agree to climb onto the table to deliver the afterbirth, I had to accept this as a reasonable compromise.

Some of what I had learned in medical school seemed to have left my memory completely. One woman who hadn't seen a doctor during her pregnancy delivered an infant daughter, whom I carried to the bassinet for the standard cleansing procedures. As I was cleaning the baby, the nurse called me back to the mother. From the vaginal opening a tiny leg protruded. I ran back to the bassinet: my first thought was that I had delivered the baby but had somehow left one leg behind! The nurse graciously brought the young doctor back to reality by gently advising him that she thought the twin was ready to deliver.

I was still learning so many things, while all around me people were still dying, and as a doctor I took every death personally. Those of us in the medical profession are generally unprepared to deal with death. We view it as some obscene shortcoming in our healing skills. This kind of professional narcissism makes it very hard to heal others. When we professionals think that we are the only ones doing the healing, we are setting ourselves up for pain and disillusionment.

I had not yet perceived the connections of spirit on the part of both patient and doctor that are involved in the total healing process. Neither could I imagine that a person could determine or know the time of his or her death. Then I met Vincente.

Vincente, a traditionalist Indian from Santo Domingo Pueblo, was in his early forties. He complained of soreness in his gut and the loss of considerable weight over the previous five months. Tests revealed that he harbored a malignant stomach tumor. We opened him up and found the tumor everywhere. There was nothing we could do.

Afterward, the incision site never healed properly, and necrotic debris continually oozed out of his belly. I tried to describe what he had and tell him about his odds, but there was no word for cancer in the Pueblos' Keres language, and I was afraid he wouldn't understand the terms in English. I said something about a kind of fire that was spreading out of control and told him that medicine, like water, did not always extinguish the flame.

Almost as if he were turning the subject away from his own mortality, he asked me how far away August 4 was. He was smiling. I thought I must be doing something wrong because Vincente didn't respond to the news of his imminent death the way I would. Instead of denying that he was dying or demanding that I do something about it, he was calmly inquiring about the most important feast day of his village.

I regretted having to say that the event was still two months away since I knew he would be dead before then. Far from the disconsolate response I had feared, he told me without hesitation that he would go home for that feast day. I said, "Fine, Vincente. I'll take you back to Santo Domingo for the ceremony," thinking with all medical certainty that he would never see that day.

But on August 4, Vincente was still alive. I drove him the thirty-five miles from the hospital to Santo Domingo in my station wagon so that he could lie down in the back. I brought dressing changes and painkilling medications with me so that I might tend to him professionally. I helped him into his home, a hot adobe house where his wife and children, other relatives, and friends came in to speak quietly with him. While he visited with these people, my family and I watched the ceremonial dances.

Here was the exotic Southwest I had envisioned. It was like walking out of the subway in New York into a living exhibit from the Museum of Natural History. The colorful clothing, the traditional dances, the tiered adobe houses with ladders propped outside were indeed as romantic as I had imagined.

But it was hard to appreciate the brilliance and grandeur of the Pueblo culture because of the overwhelming poverty of these communities. A few concrete block homes were scattered through the villages, but most were of adobe, and many had crumbling walls and corners. Families lived in one or two small rooms, and few houses had plumbing or electricity, even in the 1960s. Some of the homes had dirt floors, others wooden planks. Families carried and stored their water in fifty-gallon cans. Battery-powered radios, sewing machines, and other appliances sat outside the houses, and much of the living seemed to be a sharing of the communal outdoor spaces.

I would learn, as I lived in New Mexico, that the Pueblo culture differed in many ways from mainstream America — and not just in the absence of conveniences and consumer goods. Young Indians frequently left the pueblos and moved to the cities for school or for jobs; some established families and mortgages in the suburbs of Santa Fe or Albuquerque. Over the years, they would return to attend traditional ceremonies in their pueblos, to recharge themselves by reconnecting with their spiritual roots. As a Pueblo Indian grew older, he or she was expected to take a greater part in the rituals of the community. Parents knew that most of their sons and daughters would be drawn back there eventually by ties of many centuries. Eventually many would come back for good.

On the day I took Vincente to Santo Domingo, I saw people go into his home carrying branches and other objects that I didn't pay much attention to. Later I learned that these people were the priests of his tribe, who sprinkled corn pollen on him, brushed him with spruce branches, and blessed him with ceremonial objects.

Although Vincente was in obvious pain throughout the entire day, he never once asked for a painkilling shot. When it was time to leave, he climbed into the back of my station wagon. He did not say a great deal to his family, but he touched each one of them and waved farewell as we left. I was glad that he'd had a chance to say goodbye in a way that had meaning for him.

Back in his hospital bed that evening, Vincente announced that he was now ready to die. I downplayed his announcement, reminding him what a good day he had experienced. I told him I would see him in the morning. He said, "No. I am going to die."

In the morning I went into Vincente's room. The bed was empty. He had died during the night.

I was unprepared for an experience like this. I had been through medical school, and I knew when people were going to live and die. But this guy knew more about his own life and death than I did. He had handled the whole thing with calm dignity and certainty. That didn't make sense, and I couldn't shake the feeling of bewilderment.

I said to Bob McCormick, my colleague, "You're not going to believe this," and told him Vincente's story. He too found it astonishing, but he didn't seem as baffled as I. I think now it's because Bob was a religious man who was active in his church; he was better prepared to accept the mysterious with faith.

But Vincente's experience made an impression on me. I had a glimmer of a sense that there was something there for me to learn, but I still had no idea what that might be.

Now I know much more about the importance of ritual, the lesson I had begun to learn after watching Vincente orchestrate his farewells and his death in the way he needed to do. Ritual allows us to attach ourselves to the sacred. Sacraments permit us to see and to feel the holy. Corn pollen, sweet grass, incense, rosaries, prayer shawls—they all help us to separate the sacred from the profane or the ordinary. All these physical attachments help us to get in touch with the nontangible aspects of our spirit.

I was beginning to be ready to learn that the spirit plays as big a role in our wellness and sickness as the mind and the body do. I was, by now, becoming quite ripe for Santiago Rosetta.

Santiago, also from Santo Domingo, had been admitted to the Sante Fe Indian Hospital with congestive heart failure.

I didn't know that he was a Pueblo priest and clan chief. I only saw an old man in his seventies lying in a hospital bed with oxygen tubes in his nostrils.

Suddenly there was this beautiful smile, and he asked me, "Where did you learn to heal?"

Although I assumed my academic credentials would mean little to the old man, I responded almost by rote, rattling off my medical education, internship, and certification.

Again the beatific smile and another question: "Do you know how to *dance?*"

Somehow touched by whimsy at the old man's query, I answered that, sure, I liked to dance; and I shuffled a little at his bedside. Santiago chuckled, got out of bed, and, short of breath, began to show me his dance.

"You must be able to dance if you are to heal people," he said.

"And will you teach me your steps?" I asked, indulging the aging priest.

Santiago nodded. "Yes, I can teach you my steps, but you will have to hear your own music."

I was twenty-six years old, just out of medical school, filled with great certainties—however sorely they might be wearing away under the steady corrosiveness of pain and death. To me, at that moment in my spiritual evolution, Santiago sounded like another mystical holy man slightly removed from the realities I had to deal with. But a seed had been planted, a friendship had begun, and I later visited him many times in his home. The seeds that Santiago planted within my psyche would not sprout until I returned East.

In 1967 we left New Mexico so that I might go to Yale and study psychiatry. I had learned in Santa Fe that I wasn't willing to make a career of seeing patients seven days a week and every other night with no time to think or give patients the kind of attention I wanted to. I knew that the mind had much to do with the body's health and I was intrigued by that mystery. I have since learned that the mind will always have a mind of its own; we'll never understand it. But then I wanted to understand all that I could about the mind. Psychiatry held forth the promise of theory and explanation for the internal and eternal mysteries.

But at Yale, I encountered obstinacy as well as mystery. Several experiences showed me that I didn't belong in an urban academic setting. When I applied for a grant from Aid to Dependent Children to supplement the $4,400 a year I earned as a first-year resident, the psychiatry department was upset that the Yale salary structure had been made a matter of public display. August personages interpreted my action as a difficulty with authority that must stem from some unresolved business with my father.

Such psychiatric interpretations are designed to blunt the passion of any action, and I eventually learned not to make them. In psychiatric training, I also learned how to make and present diagnoses and, more important, when to talk and when to keep quiet. I studied the literature, the analysts, the ego-psychologists, the behaviorists, the existentialists, the geneticists, the anatomists, and the biochemists. The more I pondered the theories, the more illusory seemed the ultimate answers about the mind and body that I had hoped to find.

For a time I worked in the new facilities of the Connecticut Mental Health Center, which was situated in the "Hill" area on the fringe of New Haven's black ghetto. This was at the height of black militancy. The Bobby Seale trial had taken place in New Haven, and race riots had erupted in major cities every summer. Black leaders and groups were emerging throughout the country, and part of blacks' growing pride and self-assertion involved a strong distrust or even hatred of whites.

I was dismayed that few of my black patients stayed in treatment for any significant period of time and troubled that they saw me as an enemy. I realized they interpreted my silence during therapy as part of a power game to make them talk first. If I were going to help these people at all, I would have to do it another way.

In my search for an effective solution to the problem, I discovered community psychiatry. This technique said to me, "Get out there and use the whole system to effect change. Address the job, the boss, the school, the family, the street—use everything!" So I conducted an "after-care" clinic on Congress Avenue for people who had been discharged following a hospital stay—I conducted it in bars, on street corners, and especially in barbershops. People talked a lot easier out there too.

Nothing functions by itself, I now realized. Everything is interrelated—body, mind, and spirit. Family, community, country. Job, education, heritage, home. History, culture, religious beliefs, principles. How we put all these together in our lives makes up the unique individuals we are. My role as a therapist was to help people discover their own uniqueness in credible, healthy ways and to find what will sustain them and connect them to the larger reality of human and spiritual experience.

The New Haven race riots erupted four months after my arrival at the Mental Health Center. The center was designated an evacuation center for all the potential "crazies" who might develop as a result of this social confrontation. Interestingly, we had no psychiatric emergencies on those nights. As a matter of fact, there were actually fewer problems than usual.

Perhaps when disaster is imminent, people pull themselves together. Even the so-called crazies get it together. It is as if everybody understands that no one can tolerate madness at such explosive times.

My mentors in the psychiatry department were not pleased when I got arrested for participating in a sit-in at an abandoned city-owned building that community residents wanted to use as a drug detoxification facility—at that time there was no such facility in the city. The department once again interpreted my involvement as another manifestation of my innate problem with authority. I saw my support of the community's expression of its needs as a true demonstration of what community psychiatry was all about.

These and other experiences at Yale showed me that making a difference to people happens in the doing, not in talking about it. The seed of Santiago's wisdom had begun to sprout. He had tried to teach me that if you are going to dance, you have to move. You can't watch the dance; you can't listen to it or look at it. You have to do it to know it.

Yale was an exciting place with opportunities for taking a stand on social issues, but it wasn't the place for me. I wanted to return to the Southwest. There I could practice community psychiatry with respect for and involvement in the community's way of life.

Yet another reason for my desire to return to Indian country was that I had come to identify strongly with the Indians' struggle. I had come to see the Jewish experience as

a recapitulation of the Indian experience. You're living peace-
fully in your home and someone comes and says, "Get off
your land and give it to us or we'll kill you!" Indians were
survivors, just as my parents had been. They had seen the
handwriting on the wall in 1936 and left Germany for America. Their family members who survived were scattered
over four continents.

Leaving their home was a wrenching experience for my
relatives. My grandfather had won the German Cross in
World War I. When I visited him in Israel in 1950, he showed
it to me. He still believed that the Germany that had existed
before Hitler was a different Germany, a different experience.
He was able to distinguish Germany and the German people from the Nazis, something I'd never managed.

I grew up terrified of Germans and, at the same time, angry
at Jews and at my own Jewishness. How could all those people have been so weak and intimidated that they would just
walk into the ovens? Did this mean that Jews were by their
very nature weak and ineffectual people? I used to wonder
what I would have done if the Nazis had lined me up for
extermination. Would I have resisted? Would I have run? Was
I, too, weak?

As a boy, I would squeeze my fingernails with pliers just
to see how much pain I could stand before I screamed. I
wanted to make myself tough and show my contempt for
pain; I also wanted to hide from my fear. Yet I knew that my
self-inflicted ordeals really did not matter. Whatever pain or
suffering I could endure would never compare to what the
victims of Nazi brutality had seen and suffered.

I became preoccupied with fears of anti-Semitism. Whenever I heard people speaking German, I would feel icy claws

at my stomach. In elevators or on subways, I would eavesdrop on conversations to see if I could catch anyone making anti-Semitic comments.

None of my family ever openly discussed the concentration camp survivors. That awful time was never mentioned. Whatever had happened was too horrible to speak of ever again. I lived with the horrors and fears and guilt in my imagination.

I struggled through my adolescence complaining as little as possible. I never shared my feelings about pain, the cold, or sadness. When things got really lousy, I got through it by figuring that perhaps now I knew a small portion of the pain of other Jews. Feeling good always made me guilty for not having experienced enough sorrow.

From my efforts to define my identity as a Jew, my growing identification with Indians, and my experiences at the Connecticut Mental Health Center, I found a more certain place for myself as a doctor who could make a difference in a community. Respect for other people's experience and culture was essential before I could offer them anything from my knowledge or experience.

How different the entire history of civilization would have been if the conquerors had only viewed the conquered as having knowledge and experience to be shared. Instead victors assume the conquered have nothing to tell them because they lost, which only reinforces the belief that there is only one viewpoint, one perspective on the way—the way to truth, to knowledge, to life.

We now look to science to provide us with the answers to the Great Questions. But the answers to questions about meaning usually lie within ourselves. If we are comfortable only with answers that can be proven, we'll never really get comfortable. Science is not something to worship. We worship to acknowledge and revere the things we *don't* understand.

Interestingly, it's the physicists, like the priests and visionaries, who accept this "Uncertainty Principle." Nuclear and particle physics yield this new conviction that there are some things you can't predict. Not only does God play dice with the universe, sometimes he rolls them where you can't find them. The search for truth represents a longing, not a destination.

I have come to see clearly that those men and women who survive crises are those who have maintained a special connection to the way. They have walked their own walk with eyes open to the people and the truths around them, without discounting the walks of others. They have developed a special sense of who they are. They have supplemented the knowledge of science with a faith in the mysterious. The lesson they have imparted to me is unquestionably this: if you are going to greet the world as an equal, your feet have to be planted firmly in some unique, prideful recognition of Self. You must learn in a good way that what you are is okay. Then you can know that others are just fine too.

Our civilization has encouraged us to be independent, self-steering, goal-directed. Be your own person. Do your own thing. But sometimes we feel weak. Sometimes we feel human. At those times, we need to know that we are connected to those who came before and to those who will come after us.

This book is about medicine men and women who have helped me to learn. It is about mystery. It is about how psychiatric thinking is culture-bound. It is about the fact that neither science nor psychology has thus far provided us with a cohesive picture of the ways of human experience.

This book describes the inseparability between curing and the sense of the mystical. Healing is a powerful, culturally endorsed ritual. There is no doubt that if you trust the practitioner and if you share the same cultural myths, healing is better achieved. In the final analysis, however, I must admit that the crisis of modern life are no better alleviated by psychiatrists than by visionaries, for both attempt to provide explanations for questions that have no simple answers.

Young Indian people are coming back to reservations and communities of their forebears. They are learning their languages, their songs, their traditions. They are learning how to get connected with who they are historically and spiritually. All of us need to do the same in a way that works; we need to come back to our own truths.

I want this book to enable people to walk their own walk, wherever and whatever it may be. I do not want people to rush to the reservations to walk the Indians' walk. And I most definitely do not want them to pound on my door and insist upon walking my walk. I want each individual to seek his or her own way and to discover a personal truth.

And now the stories I learned in Indian country. I can only share these stories with you. You must set them to your own music.

Chapter 1

 BASIL

I came back to the Indian Health Service in 1970 as a civil servant, not as the commissioned officer in the U.S. Public Health Service I had been in Santa Fe.

I remained in Phoenix as Chief of Psychiatry for more than fifteen years. As someone who always had trouble with the rules and the rulers, I cannot really believe it myself. But the Indian Health Service was tolerant of me and supportive of a community-based, preventative mental health program. During my first year in Phoenix, I spent half my time at an Indian boarding school and half at the Indian Medical Center, creating a community-based program that I thought would work.

Traditionally, psychiatry has been defined as a direct service—the doctor sees individuals face to face, makes a diagnosis, prescribes treatment, and follows the patient's progress. As the only psychiatrist to cover not only the reservations spread out through Arizona, but also the Phoenix urban area, I knew there was no way I could see everyone I might be able to treat individually—and the culture itself didn't particularly fit this approach.

I decided I would teach people to help themselves. I said: "This is what I know and if you'd like to know what I know, I'd be willing to teach you. But I also want to learn what you know." So I developed a system of bringing my services to the urban and reservation communities. I got a pilot's license and flew to a different reservation once a week. I taught groups of community health workers, nurses, doctors (and their spouses), Head Start teachers, tribal jailers and inmates, and the participants in alcoholism programs. And in the process, I learned about the history, the beliefs, the lives of people in those communities.

This way I've seen far more people than I could ever have seen one on one. And I've done my job as an equal participant. I expected to learn as much as I taught; I knew these people had much to teach me. And learning from them meant gradually finding out how many things—not just about health or psychiatry—I thought I knew but didn't.

The Indian boarding school in Phoenix, where I worked half-time during my first year in Phoenix, was largely populated by youngsters sent there from their reservations for some "problem." Either they didn't get along in the public schools or their parents couldn't afford to keep them at home. For a time, our government had forced all Indian children to live in boarding schools away from home and tribal roots in an effort to make Anglo-Americans out of them. Now there are schools on most reservations, so the off-reservation boarding schools are a last resort for children or families with problems.

When I returned to the Southwest, I believed that the opportunity to work with young people would give me with the greatest opportunity to effect change. But this school, with its troubled students, proved to be too tough a place to accomplish very much. Little true learning went on because teachers and students spent most of their time struggling with each other for control of the classroom.

During my year there, I conducted a "training group" for high-school juniors and seniors. The class was billed as a "participatory learning experience," and each student received academic credit from the Social Studies Department. Fifteen students enrolled in this class, an experimental course entitled "Understanding Human Behavior."

At this time the spirit of the black revolution had just begun to reach the young Indians, and on the first day the room was full of anger. Among the pupils was Basil, who sported a headband and long braids. He was sixteen, and he didn't like me at all. It was not that Basil distrusted me; he really did not like *me*.

His opening comment to the group was that I was just another white man who had come to "lay down some more bullshit." If I had hoped to raise the consciousness of these students and get them to react, I had misunderstood the process.

Basil was not the subservient, unemotional, dependent, powerless Indian I had expected to meet. He was challenging, hostile, competitive, and the rest of the class clearly approved of what he was saying and doing to the teacher. I pulled my chair into the middle of the circle and told the students that I felt surrounded, as if I were their enemy. I complained that I did not like such treatment.

"I don't see myself as just another white man," I told them. "As a matter of fact, I had never seen myself as a white man until I came to the Southwest. I have always been a Jewish man."

I explained that I had my own history quite separate and distinct from that of any other white person they knew, and I challenged them to wait to make up their own minds about me when they knew me better.

"Just another honky scam," Basil snorted to the class. "Now they're sending some headshrinker to try to brainwash us."

"Basil," I laughed, teasing him, "you're probably Sanforized, so you're shrinkproof."

That was how the class began, and I learned something very important. If you are going to survive in Indian country, you have to learn how to deal with anger. It is laudable for teachers to tell Indian children about the past glories and noble traditions of the red man, but the truth is that what Indian children have seen for the past one hundred years of their history is not glory and greatness, but despair and disenfranchisement.

And now there was Basil hating me simply because I was white. He knew nothing of my pains, hopes, dreams, and aspirations. My being white was enough to make me eligible for his total prejudice.

Feeling Basil's uncensored anger that day was a jarring experience for me, and one of its effects was to force me to confront my own ugly racism that said all Germans were Nazis and no Christian could be trusted. Every time you actually think that you've got it together, something occurs to remind you not to take yourself so seriously. I was a well-trained, alledgedly ecumenical, nonjudgmental psychiatrist who, in dealing with someone else's prejudice, was forced once again to confront his own.

As a kid, my determining criterion for friendship was whether you would hide me in your attic if the Nazis ever came after me. That was my price for intimacy, my "Anne Frank" method of evaluating loyalty. It turned out to be a good way not to get too close to anyone. I think Jews often share a certain pride about suffering that we really don't want to give up. It's like a badge of honor: "We've suffered more than you."

I had basically settled the Christian business quite some time ago, forgiven them as a whole, and been able to become intimate friends with non-Jews. Except for Germans. Germans were always another story. Whenever I heard people speaking German, I would still quietly listen to their conversation, waiting for some anti-Semitic slur. Basil and the class of Indian students forced me to confront my own hatreds, and I have continued to struggle with those feelings ever since.

In 1983 at a tropical resort I was watching the sun set while listening to a classical music concert by the shore and reading Yaffa Eliach's *Hasidic Tales of the Holocaust*. This book, the first compilation of Hasidic stories in generations, touched me profoundly on several levels of my being through tales that once again described the reality of the horrors my family had lived through but also through stories of kindness, friendship, even laughter.

Next to me, reclining in another lounge chair, was a young woman who was also listening to the concert and watching the sun set. At the end of the performance, she leaned over and in a distinctly German accent asked if I was reading *The Holocaust*. The American mini-series of that name, she explained, had recently been shown on German television.

"No," I said, sitting up straighter (so that I might be better prepared to attack her), "these are Hasidic tales of the Holocaust. They have nothing to do with the television series. By the way," I asked, preparing to pluck an arrow from my quiver of anti-German insults, "what did you think of the television presentation?"

"I was overwhelmed," she replied in a frank and open manner. "It was, of course, all before my time. I knew very little of the period, and I must say that it has been dramatically underrepresented in German school books."

I told her that I spoke German, but rarely to Germans. However, if she were more comfortable I could converse with her in that tongue. Then, with disregard for any kind of social amenity, I told her of my great distrust, even hatred, of all Germans.

She was shocked by my vehemence. She protested that I had never been to Germany, that I had never spoken to young Germans. How could I be so angry toward a people I did not really know?

The image of my days with Basil ten years earlier flashed in my mind, but before I could examine it, I pressed on in my anger and told her a story about my parents' return to Germany in 1960. They had both come from the same small Prussian village, and they had gone back to settle some reparation business. The mayor welcomed them and presented them with flowers. As they wandered the old streets, my parents looked with tears at landmarks and memories.

They stopped at their next-door neighbors' house, and they were astonished to discover that, although quite elderly, the same people still lived there. There were tears and shouts of joy, and these elderly Christians invited my parents inside.

As they walked into the front room, my mother saw a familiar chair sitting in the corner. It was unmistakably her father's rocking chair, abandoned and forgotten in their fearful escape. When the neighbors saw that my mother recognized the chair, they explained that they had taken it from the house because the Nazis would have taken it anyway.

My mother walked out of the house and went back to the railroad station to await the next train. When it pulled out of the village, she dropped the mayor's flowers over the side. She never went back.

When I finished the story, I knew that I had experienced pain and at the same time much joy in telling it. Suffer! Writhe! I thought as I excused myself for dinner.

Just before the next evening's twilight concert, the young woman came up to me and told me that she had cried most of the night. "I cried for your pain," she said softly.

But her words made me flash in anger, so I snapped back at her, "Cry for *your* sins!"

Her firm, quiet reply was not the least bit defensive. "I am not guilty for the sins of my father."

Her words sparked an echo in my mind. It was the same thing I had said to Basil ten years earlier.

When the concert began, I retreated again into my book of Hasidic stories. This time I felt their messages about tenderness, about miracles, about human possibilities in the face of suffering. They were tales not just of horror, but of hope.

But I rejected any positive aspects of the horror stories because I had not wanted to assuage my anger. Like so many men and women, I had been replaying an old script to reexperience old suffering. I would wear it like a faded badge of honor.

When the concert ended, I made the young German woman a gift of my book of Hasidic tales. On the inside cover I inscribed, "Thank you for helping me to continue my work."

The work is never over.

Chapter 2

 HERBERT

Millions of years ago volcanic eruptions from the San Francisco peaks in north-central Arizona covered Hopiland with a hard, dry crust. Rocks eroded by age and water became mesas and canyons, some so deep that they remain dark even in sunlight.

At least one thousand years ago, an ancient farming people who called themselves the Peaceful Ones settled here after a migration that, according to their stories, lasted for thousands of years. Like others who wandered in the desert, the Hopis believed themselves to be a chosen people.

The Great Spirit, Masauwu, the guardian of this, the Fourth World, guided the Hopi to a land where settled humans could exist only by the most delicate of margins, raising nourishment in a dry and difficult land. The Hopi were instructed to stay here, and they established Oraibi and Shungopavi, the oldest continually inhabited villages in North America.

Under the inspiration of Masauwu the Hopi were divided into clans, each with its own legends and rituals that would enable them to maintain balance and harmony in this harsh land. Each generation, it was said, was to perform the rituals and ceremonies in the same manner that the Spiritual Creator had first shown them. Sternly, Masauwu decreed that the Hopi way was not to pass into the hands of others.

The Hopi religion isn't practiced just during times set aside for regular services. Like all religions are meant to do, it involves every aspect of its practitioners' lives. To follow the Hopi way is to live a life of harmony with oneself and with one's surroundings.

Anthropologists cite the Hopi way as the only indigenous belief system to have survived the Anglo-Christian conquest of North America. In the United States, the Hopi religious expression remains the sole surviving taproot of an ancient American spiritual vision.

Over the last century, however, a steadily growing number of Hopis have abandoned their ancient beliefs in favor of the white pattern of economic development. Today, most Hopi are wage earners rather than farmers.

The traditional Hopis complain that working off the reservation makes it difficult to pass on the duties of priesthood in the kiva religious societies. If the next candidate in succession for the priesthood is unavailable for the requisite practice and the exact preparation, when the old priest dies, the ceremony must simply end. And progressive elements within the Hopi have controlled the tribal government since the creation of the elected Hopi Tribal Council under the impetus of the Bureau of Indian Affairs in 1936.

Tribal traditionalists, however, continue to initiate hereditary leaders through the Bear clan. According to the Hopi way, the Creator passed the keys of survival into the hands of the village chiefs, the Kikmongwi, thousands of years ago. To lose the Hopi path here, in the planet's spiritual center, would be to sow the seeds of Earth's destruction.

Herbert Talahaftewa was of the Eagle and Forehead of the Sun clans. As spiritual leader of the two-horned society, he was responsible for the manhood initiation ceremony. I met Herbert shortly after I first came to Arizona. I had heard that he was a highly respected medicine man, a specialist in bones and joints. His services were requested by tribes as far away as the state of Washington.

Herbert was a master of manipulation of the skeleton; he also used poultices, prayers, and the application of hot stones and herbs. He cured many ailments this way, but when a problem did not respond to his methods or he knew he didn't know what to do, he told patients to see the white doctor at the white hospital. He didn't exclude other ways of looking at a problem.

Herbert was also a holy man. He had been initiated into this way by clan predecessors. Nowadays there are schools for medicine men, an idea Herbert scoffed at. To him, the power to heal was a gift. If you received it, then you could practice it and pass it on. You didn't choose to learn it; it found you.

When I was first introduced to Herbert, he was sitting at a loom weaving a ceremonial sash—for among the Hopi it is the men who weave—and wearing a baseball cap bearing with the insignia of the Caterpillar company. He had a twinkle in his eye and a cigarette dangling from a corner of his mouth, and he appeared to be in his sixties. He didn't strike me as particularly holy looking.

Herbert lived in Shungovapi, on Hopi Second Mesa. It's known as a "grandfather village," one of the most traditional

Indian villages on the reservation. Second Mesa is known for its jewelry and weaving and for Herbert's wife, Evangeline, a famous basketmaker. Herbert lived comfortably farming, weaving, and going where he was needed to heal. He lived as a religious leader who was revered in his village.

The introductions were made by a friend, who told Herbert that I was a psychiatrist, a doctor who specialized in the mind. This nugget of information did not appear to impress Herbert in any appreciable way.

When he finally turned to me, he asked, "What do you know about the mind?" His tone was one of amazement, rather than contentiousness. And I was suddenly at a loss for words. In all my training, I had never before been asked that question.

I wanted to appear competent and knowledgeable—wanted him to like me. Should I launch into a lecture about the hypothalamus, the biological determinants of behavior, neuropeptides? Somehow I did not think any of that would impress him. I could not think of a short, incisive answer.

"I guess," I replied after a painful pause, "I really don't know a whole lot about it, I mean, that can be answered briefly . . . in a short time."

Herbert smiled and went back to his weaving. He appeared to be dismissing me with his silence. (In white society, we think something is happening when people are talking. In Indian country, they know something is happening when there is silence.)

I looked around at the walls seeking some kind of solace for my awkwardness. I saw kachina carvings, pictures of children, assorted rattles. I had bungled this opportunity to become acquainted with a respected medicine man.

After what seemed to be a slice of eternity, Herbert turned to me and solemnly pronounced: "If you cannot say what you know about the mind in a short time, then you know nothing of it."

My immediate inner response was anger. This old man had just reduced all my years of education to inconsequence.

"What I know of the mind," Herbert went on, "I can tell you in one word." He paused for a moment. "Mysterious."

Mysterious. The human mind was mysterious. Herbert had looked at the question of what is mind from another perspective, from the aspect of what we don't know. It was an important lesson for me. What I know about it, he was saying, is *I don't know it*.

I wanted to learn what Herbert could teach me. I was open to him, and happily he was willing to talk, then and many times after. I call him my spiritual father. He would not make me a Hopi medicine man but he could teach me some things about the Hopi ways so I could better understand them.

In the years that we worked together after that initial meeting, Herbert often reminded me about what my studies had *not* taught me about the mind. In his opinion, schools, especially those of "higher education," attempted to teach things that were really unfathomable. Indeed, such institutions, by the very presumptuous act of pronouncing themselves "higher," supported the notion that their students could learn higher thoughts than those who had not studied there.

Herbert explained it this way: "We are like long, thin stalks of corn capped with a single gigantic ear. If the 'head' gets too big, the stalk cannot support it. Universities pay attention only to the heads and no attention to the stalks." It is the stalk that carries the spirit to the head.

According to Herbert, we have to learn from the ground up. We must be firmly rooted in the earth, because it is the real teacher. All "heads" need to be solidly connected to their "roots." To learn effectively, both the stalk and the roots must be nurtured.

During this time, in the mid 1970s, I was subjected to a series of debilitating back operations after I had suffered a badly "slipped disc," which had left my leg weak and caused my foot to drop. The surgeries had marked me with serious nerve root scarring and left a ballooning out of the lining of the spinal cord, which kept me from moving easily. I was immobilized with pain, because the drugs I had used to control the pain had stopped being effective. I had begun to prepare for a fourth operation, believing in my heart that the scalpel could cure my chronic pain by correcting the anatomic defect.

This experience of pain and what I would do to deal with it was a major watershed in my life. For the first time I was a cripple, and I wanted to be whole and mobile again. There are always two ways to look at pain: either you've got it, or it's got you. I believed that I was still athletic and strong. If only some skilled surgeon would apply the proper cut, I would be free of pain and normal again.

In retrospect, I know that I never really considered what I was doing to contribute to or intensify my pain. Basically, I was concerned only with keeping my strength up, so that when my back healed I could return to the court as a competitive racquetball player.

A week prior to the scheduled surgery, my secretary called me while I was away at a remote reservation community. She told me that Herbert was in my office and needed to see me. I spoke with him briefly and arranged to meet him in my office the following morning. That morning he asked me if I knew why he was there. I told him I didn't know what he was talking about.

Herbert didn't know why he was there either, but he had had a dream the night before last that had convinced him of his need to see me. Taking the bus to Phoenix was no small commitment for him to make in the middle of the planting season, so I knew that this visit was a true expression of how much the man cared for me.

Herbert continued talking so we could try to understand what had drawn him to visit me. On the day before his dream, he had gone to his fields to look after his first spring planting, only to discover that his seedlings had been destroyed by worms. That night he dreamed that I was standing in a shallow pit in his fields. I was covered by a grey shroud. Maggots were crawling up my legs. My mouth was wide open, but no words were coming out.

Herbert asked me again if I knew why he saw me in the dream. What was happening that would make him aware of me? I told him that I was about to be readmitted to the Mayo Clinic for surgery.

Herbert shook his head in understanding. "You are not to have this surgery. Your head is planted on a decaying stalk, my friend. It is your spirit, not your body, that needs healing."

In his own language, Herbert explained it was time for me to stand up and walk in truth. Pain doesn't go away by telling your mouth not to scream. There are some things you will no longer do, I heard him saying. The pain in your legs is telling you to stop pursuing those old messages. Lifting weights and playing competitive sports are not the only definitions of competence.

I took Herbert to the bus station. He had given me the dream, and now he had to return to the planting. I was moved by Herbert's caring, by the trouble he went to to help me. But I still wasn't ready to let go of my old dreams.

I went to the Mayo Clinic anyway, that sprawling supermarket of modern medicine. I could see in my mind the adhesions that crippled me, and I knew that if they were removed, I would be better. I knew, I believed that I could not get well without surgery.

Doctors repeated the tests. More spinal injections, more corroboration of the spinal sac deformity. I was told that I had a fifty-fifty chance for operative success.

I'm a doctor. I know that nobody goes to elective surgery with those odds. The postoperative complications alone offered the same risks as did the hoped-for cure. I still requested surgery.

A beloved friend had come to be with me. "Shmuck!" he yelled at me. "You go to elective surgery when the odds are ninety-five to five, not fifty-fifty!" He asked the surgeon what would happen without an operation. Would the back continue to deteriorate?

I had never asked that question, because I only wanted to hear that the answer was yes. That way I could fully justify placing myself in the surgeon's hands and having him "do it" to me.

The surgeon explained that my back would wear down faster than normal whether he operated or not. And, when asked if the pain could lessen without surgery, he said that with care and appropriate exercise it could. The surgeon really didn't want to operate, and my friend kept telling me I was crazy. Both of them sounded suspiciously like Herbert.

Still unconvinced but beginning to recognize the evidence, I left the clinic without surgery the next day and went to New York to see a psychiatrist, an expert in bioenergetics, with whom my friend had worked. Lying on a bed, I told the psychiatrist of my anguish, my pain, my crippledness. He imperturbably scratched his nose, and I irritably asked if he was listening to anything I was saying. He admitted that he hadn't heard much.

I wanted to leap off the bed and kill the son of a bitch but I couldn't move. "You insensitive, incompetent fraud," I screamed. "I could strangle you."

He calmly picked up a towel, twisted it, and threw it at me, motioning to me to go ahead. I became enraged. I struggled to my feet and wrapped the towel around his throat and pulled until he gasped. Only then did he push my hands away.

"Well, I'm pleased to see that you can stand," he said calmly.

Not until that moment was I aware that I was pain free! My rage had obliterated the pain. It was the most profound therapeutic intervention I'd ever had. He didn't explain or interpret my problem. He led me to express the rage I didn't know was entangled with my pain.

Symptoms—including pain—are just ways of saying something that, if you could find a way to say straighter, would make the symptoms go away. As a psychiatrist, I knew that. But I didn't know it as a patient. I thought it was something that happened to other people.

I spent the next two weeks recuperating in an upstate New York healing place where I spoke freely about frailty and fear, about Nazis and personal weaknesses. I examined the tyranny of illusions—for example, keeping my pain as another test to prove that I wasn't really afraid. No traditional healer I ever knew had to prove how tough he was.

My back pain sometimes returns, but it's never as severe as it was at that time. I can manage it; I can nurture myself with rest when I begin to feel the symptoms. I can feel it as an old friend tapping me on the back, reminding me to take care of business, to look at my life and where I'm going. Look down and get planted in truth. Listen to what you are saying to yourself.

Herbert had his own personal crisis a short time later.

The progressive leaders of the tribe had endorsed a plan for establishing indoor plumbing in the Hopi villages. They did not believe that the presence of indoor plumbing and hot water took anything away from their being Hopi.

Herbert argued that the sewer lines would disrupt invisible linkages between the kivas and between the kivas and every Hopi home. Kivas are the underground ceremonial chambers where the Kachinas, the supernatural spirits through which humankind and God communicate, live when they visit each summer. All that is sacred in the Hopi tradition is sustained in the kivas. The connections between the kivas and the Hopi had been decreed at the time of the village's creation, Herbert reminded the others. To disrupt them was to separate the heart (the kivas) from these life-sustaining veins that reached into every home on the mesa.

Herbert said that if the connections were broken by this seduction of convenience, it would signal the destruction of the Hopis' special covenant with the Creator. You don't exchange lifelines for sewage disposal. To him, it was that simple.

The village went ahead with the sewer project. So Herbert took another kind of action—he lay down in front of the bulldozer. The construction crew threatened to roll over him, but Herbert wouldn't move. They said they would seek an injunction from Tribal Court and then return. There were no statutory precedents relating to invisible underground connections.

Soon after the encounter, Herbert had a heart attack while in the kiva. He had been fasting and preparing for a ceremony when he simply keeled over. He was over seventy years old. One of the other participants revived Herbert with cardiopulmonary resuscitation. After a brief hospitalization, he was discharged.

Although less active, he still did carpentry work around the house. He was consumed with concern that with white people, Bahaanas, forcing their way into their sacred land, many Hopis would abandon their difficult way. Prophecy had told him that if the Hopi no longer respected their traditions, the land would shrink to nothing.

To Herbert and others, these ancient prophecies were coming true. Fewer young Hopis were passing through the final initiation in which they were given their true Hopi names—not because they didn't want to, but because there were few left who could perform the ceremony properly.

Herbert spent more time alone in the house. He was a traditional chief whose life had been restored in the kiva, and everyone looked at him now with a mixture of awe and fear. He had always been a powerful figure, but his death and rebirth experience had given him a ghostlike quality. Herbert too felt the distance, and we talked about it.

Then one day, as suddenly as it had happened in the kiva, Herbert died from a massive blood clot to his lungs.

I visit his gravesite regularly. It sits below the mesa, and like the others it's covered with sand, stones, and pieces of pottery. The Hopi don't encourage visitors to their cemeteries. When I go to see Herbert, I don't stay long. I tell him I'm feeling better.

In the distance, the silence is broken by the noise of the sewerline machinery.

Chapter 3

 PROUD MARY

O̶ne day as I was leaving Dilkon, a remote Navajo
reservation town just off Arizona Highway 87, I saw a pretty,
long-haired young woman hitchhiking. As the father of three
daughters, I am very uneasy about female hitchhikers. Too
many of them end up violated.

She seemed to be intent upon leaving Dilkon, which is
situated halfway between the Hopi Second Mesa villages and
the city of Winslow. In the huge expanses of land that make
up Arizona's Indian reservations, villages are many miles
apart. There is only one major road through this part of this
reservation, and the only place it leads is to Winslow, which
I had to pass through on my way back to Phoenix. She had
to be going my way.

"Hop in," I told her as I pulled my van over.

She accepted my hospitality without a word. Once inside
the van, she looked very young, and I felt good that I had
stopped for her. Her features were not finely chiseled in the
classic Roman way, but she was pretty in a softer, less angu-
lar way. She wiped her nose on her sleeve, and I pointed to
the box of tissues that I always kept in the van.

"I only want a ride from you," she said sharply. "Nothing else."

Jeez, I save this young woman from a fate worse than death, and in return I get snarls instead of appreciation. After a few more miles of silence, she apparently decided to make herself even clearer.

"If I had a choice," she stated bluntly, "I wouldn't have taken a ride from you or from any white man."

You didn't have to be a psychiatrist to see that she was troubled. I would conveniently serve as the immediate scapegoat—I'd been in Indian country long enough to play that scene patiently.

"The white man destroyed this place of harmony," she continued. "They always took more than they needed." On and on. Not at all a participatory conversation. She was very bright.

When she stopped her invective, I didn't feel as if I had anything to say—or for that matter anything to apologize for. I just nodded so she would know I heard her.

At Winslow, I pulled the van in in front of a cafe. After a few minutes of maintaining a solitary vigil in the van, she joined me inside.

"I agree with some of your ideas," I told her, now that she seemed willing to listen because she wanted to eat. "But I have worked here long enough to know that it isn't only the white people whose values have become distorted. Look at your reservation," I challenged. "It's littered with broken glass, tin cans, garbage. You've lost the path too. Being out of balance, existing in disharmony, is not a disease that favors one color of skin."

It was my turn now, and I was warming to the occasion.

Perhaps she was only quiet because she was eating her hamburger, but I took advantage of the fact that she was chewing on her sandwich and not on me.

"All people are interested in the same things," I waxed on. "We all want a place to sleep, a family, and children to give at least as much to as we ourselves have been given. These basic desires really make us all the same."

The young Navajo's response to my pontification was to belch and walk out of the cafe. I paid the tab, then joined her back in the van. If my conversation was not acceptable, if my skin color was not desirable, at least my wheels were still considered necessary. As we headed out of Winslow, she asked me what I did for a living.

"I am an interpreter of dreams," I replied.

Her response: "Blow it out your ass."

The remainder of the ride went more quickly though the conversation was no warmer. I dropped her off at a convenience market inside the Phoenix city limits and waved goodbye.

Another embittered young Indian, wrapped in anger and confusion.

Some weeks later, a "Mary" left a number with my secretary. I didn't recognize the name, but when I returned the call, the voice at the other end of the line asked me to remember her.

"Remind me."

"I liked the ride down from Dilkon."

Aha! The voice came back to me. So my bright but bitter passenger was named Mary. I truly was surprised to hear from her but delighted that she wished to talk to me about her career plans.

"How about lunch sometime next week?" I offered.

"That would be wonderful," she accepted.

We continued our lunches for two years. Mary told me her story, and I told her mine.

As a child, Mary had sat with her oldest sister night after night waiting for their mother to come home. Mama had grown tired of waiting for Daddy to come home from the tavern, so she joined him and they both drank. Eventually, both would be driven home in the back of some relative's pickup truck. Mary excused her mother: perhaps she really had no choice. With twelve children to support and unable to change her husband's behavior, she gave up too.

It is impossible to talk about Indians without talking about alcoholism. Some theorists say that the 50-to-90-percent rate of alcoholism on the reservations results from a genetic proclivity to metabolize alcohol in a damaging way. I see it differently.

Drinking is another way to suckle nurturance, I told Mary. Nobody makes it alone in the world; we all need something to depend on. If beliefs and traditions don't provide good ways to meet our needs for dependency, we become vulnerable and seek other, more destructive sources of nurture.

Many Indians have been separated from what they believe in by the domination of another culture and by poverty and discrimination. When individuals find little to sustain them in being Indian, the bottle helps them escape the reality.

Once Indians used alcohol as a sacrament in specific rituals, but when a sacrament is misused, it destroys the user. Whether this suicidal process goes slowly or fast, I told Mary, it stems from a simple desire to be heard and an inability to find anyone to listen. If you can discover ways of talking about your feelings more directly to someone you like and believe in, most symptoms disappear—except for the damage done to the body in the meantime.

Mary's father had been found frozen to death in a ditch, another alcoholic death. Her mother continued to drink alone. When Mary was four, she and her siblings were split up, and she was placed in an off-reservation home. This was not an uncommon way for large Indian families to manage when there just wasn't enough money to feed everyone.

Mary's earliest recollections of her new white family included picnics and church. She loved her new life, even though she had readily perceived that she was different from everyone else in her new environment. Church reassured Mary that if she believed, sooner or later she would become "whitesome and delightsome." Mary had convinced herself that as she grew older, her skin would turn paler.

It never happened, and by thirteen she had become a sullen management problem. Mary would get into fights with teachers as well as classmates. She would dare those in authority to do something to her.

In one sense, Mary's trouble stemmed from the ordinary questions of the adolescent in search of an identity: Who am I? What do I really believe in? Mary's queries were complicated by the fact that she was not firmly planted in any unique sense of self. She was unsure of who she was ethnically or where her true home was.

Mary was angry at her white mother for adopting her. She was angry with her Navajo mother for abandoning her. She had completely lost touch with her family on the reservation. As she searched for herself in this conflicting background, her schoolwork deteriorated and she began to steal from her adoptive parents.

When Mary declared that she wanted to go to Indian boarding school, her social worker thought that the Indian identification might be helpful. Her adoptive parents agreed, for she had now exceeded their capacity to deal with her.

At the school, Mary discovered other young Indians who had been sent there from extreme poverty, from alcoholic abuse, from non-English-speaking families, from problems in public schools. They came from a variety of tribes and from diverse backgrounds. What most of them had in common was some problem fitting in where they had been.

Indian boarding schools are frequently understaffed and exhibit a critically low morale. Consequently, the teachers do not teach a lot; the students do not learn a lot; and very little behavior is controlled or constructively modified. Mary had been a scholastic star before her troubled teens had set in motion her downhill slide. In the boarding school she became an academic jewel.

But her identity struggle just became more complicated. The teachers loved her, but Mary did not fit in with the other students. She looked like the rest of them, but she was verbally proficient while most of the others were sullen and silent. Mary could not find happiness in a place where her peers either ignored or ridiculed her.

One day during her first year in boarding school, Mary went shopping in a nearby mall. In a drugstore, she bent down to hold a tin of shoe polish next to her boots to see if the colors matched. The store manager appeared and asked her if she intended to steal the shoe polish. Mary answered unhesitatingly that she was just matching the colors, but he was convinced that she was lying. He next accused her of stealing the items in her shopping bag that she had bought from the department store next door.

Even after the department store personnel verified that Mary had paid for the items, the drugstore manager wasn't satisfied. His clear prejudice wouldn't relent. He told Mary that even if she didn't steal the shoe polish, he knew she was thinking about it. Officiously, he ushered her out the back door, telling her not to come back.

Mary cried with rage, first at him, then at whites. She beat trees, cursed, turned over garbage cans, scrubbed her room to expend some of the seemingly endless rage held in from a lifetime of not belonging.

Then she started a chapter of a militant Indian organization. Her identity was becoming clear—she knew she was Indian. However she was seen by the world, she would flaunt her Indianness, her way. She got buttons, emblems, and bumper stickers. She sent away for posters of American Indian chiefs and sold them at the school.

It doesn't really matter how you get your anger out, only that you get it out. For Mary, anger turned out to be the catalyst to finding the long-needed answer to the question, "Who am I?"

At eighteen, after finishing school, Mary hitchhiked to an Indian commune in California where the people called her "Proud Mary" after the Creedence Clearwater Revival's popular song. At that time, in the mid-seventies, large numbers of young Indians were struggling with what it meant to be Indian. From their political movement, spiritual communities arose, where the young studied the elders' stories, dances, and cosmology. During her time in the commune,

Mary contacted a social worker who helped her locate her biological family.

Mary returned to Dilkon, hitchhiking again. At the town's only store she asked if they knew of her family. In halting English, they pointed out the direction.

Mary walked two miles to a compound comprised of a wooden house, a separate earth and wood hogan, and surrounding corrals. She walked past the chickens, dogs, and bloody sheepskins to approach an old woman sitting in front of the house. This old woman could be her mother. Mary was overwhelmed with that awareness. She didn't know how she would react.

Mary waved at the woman and tried to converse. There was no response, except for a shrug of the shoulders. The old woman understood no English.

Another woman came into the compound with a group of children. Luckily they all spoke English. After a few minutes of conversation, it became clear that this was Mary's sister, together with her nieces and nephews. The two sisters hugged and cried.

In the next hours she learned that her other brothers and sisters had returned home after their first years in foster placement. Only Mary had been adopted.

The family told Mary's mother in Navajo that this stranger was her youngest daughter, the little girl she had given away long ago. But no matter how many ways they told her, the woman didn't remember having another child. The years of alcohol, poverty, and pain had taken their toll on her mind.

What Mary had hoped to get from her mother, a sense of home and belonging, her mother could no longer give. But

Mary could get those things from the rest of her family, who eagerly welcomed her back. Her brothers and sisters wanted to sponsor a welcoming-home ceremony. Mary was overjoyed by the prospect. This was the fulfillment of her search for a place where she belonged.

The ritual of the ceremony helped to heal the rift, the many lost years that Mary had suffered. Now she could begin to know her self, to be whole. By the time I met Mary, she had learned that you can have your feet planted in more than one place and still know who you are.

Navajo medicine men and women use ritual to help restore mental and physical health. They do not reject Western medical or psychological concepts—they only see them as limited. They see the universe as filled with many enormously powerful forces, all of which hold the potential for good and evil. If, for some reason, the balance between good and evil is upset, people get sick. You have to keep in balance if you want to stay healthy.

Mental health is the same way. It can be described as having your head, mouth, and heart in a straight alignment. Mental health happens when what you believe in your heart is the same as what you say with your mouth. You are mentally healthy when what you feel is something you also believe. When the alignment isn't straight, when the mouth doesn't say what the heart feels or when the head knows something the heart doesn't choose to acknowledge, then sooner or later you will get sick.

The traditional Navajo ceremony that Mary's family held to welcome her back helped to restore Mary's balance—and theirs too. This was the way in which they could come together again and Mary could become whole.

The ceremony was held in a hogan. Mary was frightened that she would make mistakes and not be able to repeat exactly the words of the prayers. Her sister helped her learn her part in the ritual.

The medicine man knew every word for the entire ceremony in exactly the right order, each line with its appropriate melody. As he sang, he sprinkled multicolored sands on the ground with movements of his thumb and forefinger, creating what many believe to be the greatest folk art on this continent.

Mary stared at the sand painting in awe. It depicted a Navajo legend about a child who was lost to the tribe, but who returned in another form. The medicine man asked Mary to sit in the middle of the painting. Now she could actually mingle with the heroic figures and absorb their strength.

The medicine man tied feathers and spruce on Mary and placed stone and wooden fetishes, holy objects, on her. He twirled a wooden noisemaker and made a huge roar. Mary felt the breeze from this instrument as if it were blowing her old confused and angry self away.

The medicine man gave her a pipe filled with sweet tobacco. He smoked it; she smoked it; and they blew clouds of tobacco smoke over themselves and toward the sky. For everyone, the atmosphere was charged with feeling.

This was how Mary's odyssey ended. She could like flush toilets, watch television, become well educated, and still be Navajo. She could perceive the world as angry and hostile or as nurturing and sustaining. She had the choice. She could always connect with the things that really mattered. Mary now works among her Navajo people as a health professional.

When we met, Mary was filled with anger at her own exploitation, then anger at white people. She finally gave up the anger. All of what she was served to remind her not to close her eyes to other realities. By hearing all the voices within herself, Mary made a new friend.

Mary kept the parts of herself in alignment by remembering the words sung in her ceremony:

Happily—may you walk with God—
Happily—may you walk—
Happily—may you feel light within—
Happily—with feeling may you walk—
Happily—may you walk with God.

All of us need to connect with authentic paths home.

Chapter 4

 MILTON AND ERICH

Patty had been referred to me from the hospital's emergency room with "self-inflicted burns." She sat in my office staring at her hands, her straight, shoulder-length hair covering her face like a shroud. She looked about twelve years old but she was nineteen, and four months pregnant. Her husband had brought her to the emergency room after he had found her sticking lighted matches into her navel.

Patty told me that a hummingbird had flown into her bedroom window and had somehow gotten stuck behind the dresser mirror. In trying to escape, the hummingbird had broken its neck. She was convinced that her unborn baby now had a broken neck too. She further believed that it was trying to get out of her body. If the baby remained inside of her, it would kill her. She had been trying to burn it out of her before it did her in.

Patty had not been drinking; nor was she on drugs. I hospitalized her because she was delusional.

From her records, I learned Patty's parents had died in a house fire when she was nine years old. Patty's pregnant sister had been awakened by the smoke, and she had managed to get the rest of the children out of the house before she returned to attempt to rescue their parents. The sister had been overcome by smoke and falling debris, and she also died. Patty's earliest memory was seeing her sister's belly pop open as her body was roasted.

Patty was sent to an Indian boarding school with her younger brother. Eight months later he was dead from a bee sting that had caused his windpipe to swell shut.

Patty left the school when she was thirteen and pregnant. She went to live with the boy's family, and after the birth of the child, his parents adopted it. Patty eventually moved out of the home and married someone else.

By sixteen, she was an abused wife. At least twice her husband was jailed for beating her. Following each of those severe beatings, she miscarried.

For Patty, everything that was lovable was eventually taken from her. If you believe that sooner or later some disaster is going to befall you, then the only control you have in that situation is to make it happen at your time, rather than to wait. That's why she stuck the matches into herself in the first place.

She had believed her baby would die. Another thing she loved would be taken from her. So she tried to make it happen her way and in her time. It was the only choice for her; she could never have given birth and then given the child up.

Now Patty's twenty-one-year-old husband was unemployed. He showed up in my office drunk one day, and he never returned. Patty miscarried while she was in the hospital. Slowly she began to get better.

She told me that she dreamed that snakes were coming out of blisters on the palms of her hands. Sometimes dozens of snakes would come out at once. When the blisters burst, the snakes would fall out and writhe about on her body. She would awaken from the sound of her own screaming.

Death was always around her, she said. Everything that she touched would die. She believed that she had some terrible power to attract death.

Just after the miscarriage, Patty feared that there might still be a piece of her baby inside of her, "turning into shit, to kill me." She tried burning holes in her belly again, to get the shit out.

I told her she wasn't trying hard enough to get her shit-baby out. I said that she must eat vegetables and high-fiber food to remove it. Then I bent over the broccoli on her lunch tray and spoke to it. I told it to cleanse Patty's insides with its fuzzy brush head. She ate it, and I prescribed a powerful laxative. She suffered from diarrhea and cramping, but when it was all over, she started to get well.

Milton

I understood this kind of stuff better after I had discovered Milton Erickson. His basic tools were always whatever the patient gave him, not just what he had learned in medical school. Erickson firmly believed that the doctor and the patient must share the same language and symbols and that they must together trust the unconscious. The doctor was only the guide as the patient walked his or her walk.

Milton Erickson was a maverick psychiatrist whose strategy was never to be restrictive and always to do the unexpected. A doctor did not have to know everything about his or her patients to be able to penetrate into the unconscious. In the proper learning environment, change could occur suddenly. One had to sneak into the unconscious mind with a message that it could hear: through indifference that triggers anger, through talking to broccoli, through religious or tribal ritual.

He knew that not everything can be explained. What's important in therapy is not direct interpretation; it's finding a way to get the person to pay attention. Erickson spoke in metaphors, in stories.

It has been my observation that many therapists avoid intervention with unconscious material because it makes treatment seem so simple. It is also rather frightening to assume that much responsibility, to trust your intuition along with your education.

Erickson wasn't afraid. He showed us that you have to use *all* of your healing skills if you want to do the work well. A healer is simply someone who helps a person confront opposing forces within him- or herself to promote health. Healing is accomplished whenever the needs of such opposing forces are successfully negotiated.

Erickson once said that the most important teacher he ever had was polio. As a child he was crippled, tone deaf, and color blind. He was also dyslexic. He taught himself to distinguish between the number "3" and the letter "M" because the three was "sitting" and the M was "standing."

Erickson insisted that you always make the best of the cards that life has dealt you. All people have things from their own experiences that they might use to see events and feelings more clearly. You are like your fingerprint—unique. There will never again be another you.

I had not learned of Erickson's theories at Yale. Even though at least twenty books have been written by or about

Erickson, his techniques were not taught there. They still aren't studied in most medical schools, now that psychiatry is moving toward a more "medical" approach that believes everything can be explained by biochemistry.

About a year before his death I met Erickson himself.

I had read some of his writings, and I knew that he understood what I was seeing and feeling in my work with the Indians. I was excited to meet this master who had already discovered what I was learning: to make changes, everyone— doctor and patient—must find his or her own unique way to fuel the creative unconscious.

Milton Erickson was in his late seventies when we met. I giggled aloud as I got my first look at his office, located behind his home in Phoenix. This rectangular add-on was decorated in vintage chrome and vinyl bus depot style. There were assorted ill-matched chairs, two-headed dolls, bones, dried fish, coconut skull with electric eyes. Erickson's wife, Betty, helped him into the study in his wheelchair. He was dressed completely in purple, the only color he could see. He sat there like an elf, a crooked smile betraying the weaker side of his body.

Milton looked at me, and I knew that my own smile of appreciation and excitement had given me away.

He leaned forward from his wheelchair and reached for a rock-sized piece of turquoise ore. For several moments he struggled with the task of picking up the rock. The process was obviously costing him a great deal of effort. I was spellbound, entranced with the silent drama of Erickson picking up a rock.

Then, while he looked at me and I looked back at him, he threw the rock directly at my crotch. For a moment I thought that I would be leaving the man's office with a high-pitched voice. Before I could react, the "rock" landed on me. It was a piece of foam rubber.

Erickson chortled and, in his Viking godfather voice, cautioned me: "Not everything you see is what you see it as. It is only how you see it at the moment."

Or did he say that how you saw it at the moment was really the way it was?

I was confused, but I sat there under his spell. Erickson was like a medicine man in his hogan. He was a storyteller capable of spinning magic.

Sometimes he would have his patients make pilgrimages to mountaintops, telling them to write down what they had seen and experienced during the climb. On occasion he prescribed ordeals, challenges that led people face to face with their monsters, their fears. These are the rites of passage into selfhood that many adults have never made. Indians have such a spiritual tradition, the vision quest. The purpose is to go to a quiet, isolated place and in solitude and readiness open oneself to receive what the mind wants to tell. The vision quest, like psychotherapy, is a transforming ritual.

Erickson could be a clown or a magician. He often used secret words, even fetishes such as masks and dolls. In Zuni legends, fetishes, usually carvings of animals in stone or shell, contain a spirit and will provide supernatural assistance to the owner. We use the same term in psychiatry to describe an object that a person has invested with magical, often sexual, powers. Clearly, such objects, in whatever way they become fetishes, hold a key to our unconscious minds.

· Erickson never made a direct interpretation of symbols like fetishes or dreams. He was a master of enabling people to see their own symbols, to establish a pipeline into their own unconscious selves. He called this "strategic therapy," and like a skilled medicine man he helped his patients to maintain their own genuine, true connection to their centers.

Direct interpretations, Erickson argued, were an assault on the unconscious. The unconscious could find more ways to resist hearing something than you could find ways to say it. The therapist must approach the unconscious indirectly, even seductively, inviting it to reveal itself.

Repeatedly, Erickson emphasized that each individual was unique. Differences were to be treasured.

After our marvelous day-long session, I saw him one last time to give him a special gift, a Hopi Sun kachina, the messenger of enlightenment. A Kachina is a spirit, represented by dancers in Hopi ceremonies. Hopis teach their children about the spirits through the use of kachina dolls carved from the root of the cottonwood tree and painted to resemble the dancers. The Indians have many ways of keeping their centers visible.

At that last visit, Erickson and I sat together in his living room. The floor was virtually covered with Seri Indian carvings, lustrous heavy ironwood animals produced by a Mexican tribe along the Sea of Cortez. Before I left, he asked me to get him a leather pouch that was hanging on the door. It was a medicine bundle, the kind in which an Indian healer carries his or her most powerful tools. He unwrapped a gazing crystal and held it lovingly as I said goodbye.

Milton Erickson was a dancing healer. Herbert would have understood him, and Santiago would have applauded his dance.

Erich

A couple of months after Erickson died in 1980, another mentor, Erich Fromm, passed away. I wondered about the coincidence. Two months after Fromm's death, Mt. St. Helen's in Washington state erupted. Clearly, it was a season of change.

Herbert once told me that there would come a time when the seasons would change drastically. Summers would become unusually dry and winters would bring floods. There would be earthquakes and upheavals. Mt. St. Helen's, he would say, was a potent sign that the Earth was tired of its defacement by humankind. (Interestingly, the volcano obliterated a body of water at its base called Spirit Lake.)

The concern of Herbert and the other Indian traditionalists for the earth's rebellion was of long standing. In 1944, the BIA Hopi Agency had received inquiries from oil companies and other energy corporations about exploration leases for mineral deposits in Hopi land. At that time, the traditional religious leaders had written a letter to President Harry S. Truman affirming their position:

> This land was laid out for us by our Great Spirit. . . . It is given to the Hopi People, the task to guard this land. Not by force of arms . . . but by humble prayers, by obedience to our traditional and religious instructions. . . . This land is not for leasing or for sale. . . . Land is sacred and if the land is abused, the sacredness of the Hopi life will disappear and all other life as well. . . . Hopis are caretakers for all of the world.

Their case was rejected by a federal district court in Arizona, and the court decision was soon followed by the arrival of the oil companies, the explosions, and the digging for coal. According to Hopi prophecy, after such a violation of the earth, the state of order and harmony all over this planet would crumble. When the people couldn't follow the way anymore, then the Great Spirit would take the power into its own hands.

Erich Fromm would have understood this belief perfectly.

I liked Fromm and identified with him. He was a German Jewish refugee to the United States, a psychologist, and a mystic who once studied Kabbala with the foremost scholar of Jewish mysticism, Gershom Scholem.

Fromm was a founder of SANE, Committee for a Sane Nuclear Policy, an organization that warned of the danger of nuclear weapons. Like the Hopis, he feared that the earth and humankind were headed toward psychological and ecological disaster. In an age dominated by technology and consumerism, Fromm said, we are in danger of growing to feel more and more insignificant and uncertain about the meaningfulness of life. Fromm reached the simplest of conclusions: we must live by love. It was the only sane way to save ourselves from meaninglessness.

Once, I must admit, I viewed certain of these concepts as marshmallow fluff. But as I became a healer, I saw that people need love and a shared sense of spirit if they are to find a place to secure themselves in peace and belonging.

Fromm was a revolutionary in his own right. Once a disciple of Freud, he shed his mentor's sex-explains-everything libido theory, because he thought it a terribly confining position that didn't help us understand families and societies. Fromm admonished that society didn't place much importance on what was good for humankind. As a matter of fact, what was *bad* for humans did not make a whole lot of difference in contemporary thinking either. Toxic wastes in earth and air are the byproducts of the same genius that fashioned the labor-saving technology that we call progress.

The exploitation of humankind and nature renders us all out of touch with our feelings and basic needs, Fromm believed. Our technological genius entraps us and transforms us into machines. People hide behind masks of success. Though more of us have opportunities to amass wealth and comforts, we hide the truth of our depressions, annoyances, and unhappinesses.

Most people, Fromm thought, become co-opted by the demands of industrialized society for more production, more consumption, and more progress. But more progress in economy and technology does not mean more progress in people's search for meaning. The progress we have achieved is being directed away from the real spiritual and emotional betterment of people to an evil inner desert.

Fromm had no patience, however, with those who rush to embrace mystical philosophies to answer these dilemmas. He saw most of those as pure fakery and con-artistry, just more slick commercialism and salesmanship. Not everybody who said they had found the way really had. Using modern business methods, he believed, one could sell anything.

There was nothing fluffy about Fromm. He looked fearlessly at some of the truths organized religions and the healing professions often dodge.

Fromm is another healer who can help us get back on the path to pursue our vision quest.

Chapter 5

 **THE CHURCH
OF FATHER PEYOTE**

The first time I attended the church of Father Peyote,
I got quite sick—and I was only sitting outside listening to
the music. They passed some tea around. I tried it and became
violently ill.

I thought that was the end of my relationship with Father
Peyote. There was no way that I would sit up all night just
to get sick. On that first visit to a Native American Church
meeting in 1965, I did not realize that the process it offered
was not to be taken lightly. It took me ten years to make a
return visit, but now the church has become a place of healing and enlightenment for me.

To the believer, peyote constitutes a sacrament, not a drug.
Peyote has absolutely no recreational aspects for the church
participants. You must come to peyote as to truth, in an attitude of worship.

Let me explain at the outset that in matters of the Peyote
Church, I am a guest who has come to dinner; that does not
make me an expert on the entire family. I know what I have
seen, and there is much I don't know. I go as a fellow
traveler. I don't bring friends to observe the colorful ritual.

This is a sacred time to me and to every other participant in the service.

The most spiritual place I know is the tipi of the Peyote Church. I used to go to synagogue on the high Jewish holidays, but I can no longer feel the presence of the spirit in a group larger than forty.

Indians have a very different concept of where you worship. The whole Earth is the temple. Any place you stand is a church. The tipi is a nestling enclosure on the Earth Mother's breast, a place of sharing among a small group. Here each can worship at his or her own time, as the heart directs, in his or her own language.

I sing my Jewish songs in the tipi, and I wear my father's prayer shawl, the one he wore at his bar mitzvah in Germany. My Indian friends say that it does not matter in what language you sing; there are always at least two people who understand—you and the Creator.

The first time I sat before the coals in the tipi, I saw crematorium ashes. I do not see them as such anymore. I have allowed myself to become liberated. I understand that I am flawed and imperfect, so it's okay to feel small and weak. I am freer of the domination of those fears.

The more you work with the mind, the more you realize you can't know it. The more you seek to touch your spirit, the more you realize that you must enter some altered state of consciousness to burst free of the conventional limitations of flesh and rationality. This is what the Peyote Church is about.

I became interested in returning to the Peyote Church after I met a Road Man—a Native American Church leader, the "one who shows the road"—who asked me where I got my power to heal. I had heard that question before, so I smiled and answered, "I am still learning how to dance."

The Road Man smiled too. He told me that his healing power came through the sacrament peyote. "Oh," I said, a bit dubious. "I participated in a peyote meeting once and it felt more like a punishment than a gift."

He laughed and said that peyote's gift really depended on how you came to it. If you were a skeptic and approached it with fear, peyote would not reveal itself. He assured me that I could learn to receive the gift. This is a man I have since come to respect; we have taken each other as brothers.

I once provided testimony in support of passage of the Native American Religious Freedoms Act. From a psychological perspective, I testified, if the Native American Church did not exist, it would have to be created. I believe the church is one of the most important pan-Indian movements in this country. It offers a credible connection to something uniquely Indian. It is political, cultural, and spiritual—a source of pride, power, and psychological health.

The Native American Religious Freedoms Act was signed into law by President Jimmy Carter in 1978, but it has not yet been fully implemented. Although the powerful hallucinogen peyote is illegal to possess or use, the law allows Indians to consume it as a sacrament in the Native American Church, because of its traditional role in Indian religious beliefs. However, some states do not exempt church members from prosecution if they buy or sell it.

There is evidence of the ritual consumption of peyote as a sacrament by priests for more than sixteen hundred years, as far back as the Mayans. Legends tell that the sacred quality of peyote was revealed to a woman. One version says that a pregnant woman, lost from her band, wandering and alone, sick and weak, gave birth to a child. She was sustained by a vision that told her to eat the plant that was growing beside her. The plant was to be life and blessing for her and her people. She regained her strength, found her band, and shared the blessing.

The Navajo peyotists say that during the creation, it was the sacrament peyote that gave life, breath, and movement to Rainbow Woman, their birth-mother.

The Native American Church, as it is practiced in Arizona today, is only one hundred years old. It is commonly held that the faith came to the Oklahoma territory a century ago through Quanah Parker, a Comanche Indian leader. While living with his white mother's family in Texas, Quanah fell ill. When the doctors could not help him, the family called in an Indian healer; she cured Quanah with the help of songs and a bitter tea.

When Quanah recovered, the woman told him that the magical tea must never be taken for its own sake. It must be taken as a sacrament, with ceremony and respect. The medicine, peyote, came from the buttons that grow on the mescal cactus, and it was to be used for prayer, understanding, and healing—it was a sacred thing.

The healer showed Quanah the way to the sacred cactus and told him that it must be stalked like one stalks a deer—with respect. No one should wear the red mescal beads except during the ceremony and because woman first brought peyote to the earth, woman must always have a place in the ritual. She brought him to the meeting fireplace where he learned the ceremony.

When a healthy and fully recovered Quanah returned to

Oklahoma, it was a time of seething Indian discontent. The tribes were chafing under the confines of a neocolonial federal Indian policy that followed the bloody wars throughout the Southwest and Great Plains that decimated so many tribes. The Plains tribes were falling apart; the life-sustaining buffalo were disappearing.

Christian churches were springing up everywhere among the Indians. Their central myths were already familiar through traditional Indian beliefs. Virgin births, saviors, miracles, healings, and raising people from the dead already made sense, and the church promised salvation.

Also at this time Wovoka, a Paiute, introduced to the Plains tribes a new amalgamation of tribal religions and Christian elements called the Ghost Dance. The Ghost Dance was based on a hatred of whites and a hope of doing away with them to bring back the old Indian ways. Dancers wore cotton or buckskin shirts painted with "bulletproof" designs to protect the wearer. The vests didn't work, but the movement hasn't failed. Feelings against whites still bring all Indians together. The Ghost Dance is undergoing resurgence, as are so many traditional Indian ways.

Into this atmosphere Quanah brought the sacrament peyote back to his Comanche tribe. A vision at the holy mountain near present-day Cache, Oklahoma, ordered him to bring this sacrament to his people to perpetuate the ways he had been taught. Quanah brought the beads and the sash worn by the Peyote Chief, called the Road Man. He also brought the elements of the peyote ceremony: fire and cedar incense, the water drum, the peyote fans, the staff, the gourd rattle, and the smoking of sweet tobacco and peyote.

The peyote religion spread throughout the Indian world, each tribe adding its own variations. The Christian churches and government agents argued against it as the way of the Devil that transformed their Indian flocks into drug-crazed savages. But many of the Indians saw it as something of their own, a way to the spirit. The Navajo were introduced to peyote in the early 1900s, probably through students who were initiated in boarding schools. Soon tribes from east to west were holding peyote ceremonies.

This uniquely pan-Indian religion today may have as many as 300,000 participants. Many observers have found it to be the single most effective program to deal with the problem of Indian alcoholism.

The Native American Church has members from nearly every tribe on the North American continent. It sometimes incorporates Christian symbology in its rituals, yet it expresses the ideals of the older traditions: each individual is a part of the harmonious creation of the universe. With all things we are as brothers and sisters and must live together in harmony and peace. The Earth Mother must be treated with respect and gratitude.

The members of the Native American Church are essentially universalists, regarding all religions as basically good and variations on the same theme. They stress humility, faith, and love toward all and believe that a man or woman trying to function alone is weak. All must seek the Creator's guidance for true strength and redemption. Peyote offers the communicant a method of establishing contact with the Creator.

I liked the Road Man I met. He was not a salesman, just a believer. We talked about treatment failures as well as successes. He said undefensively that his failures reminded him that he was just one small cog in a much bigger machine. The mysterious was unfathomable. I knew in my heart that I was more ready now to participate in Father Peyote's church than I had been before. The Road Man invited me to a service.

We met at the tipi at dusk for a ceremony that would last until sunrise. In the enclosing darkness, people talked in small groups, and other than the Road Man, I knew no one. Then at nightfall we lined up in front of the huge tipi, which held more than thirty people around a central fire. I felt like a traveler to another place and time.

The taking of the awesome, psychodynamically powerful drug still frightened me a little. But I went to the meeting with a positive attitude, and the Road Man had reassured me that it would take care of itself. He respected the power of peyote and he had never seen problems. He explained that everyone had come together for the purpose of enlightenment.

It was time. We walked around the tipi while the Road Man chanted. Then we entered, following the Road Man through a flap opening on the east side where the sun's first rays would strike. The Road Man, also called the chief, sat at the west end, opposite the tipi opening. On the Road Man's right was the man who "carried drum"; on his left, the sponsors of the meeting. The other participants all sat on the earth floor on blankets, strips of carpet, or pillows. Because of my back problem, I had brought a small beach chair; afterward some called me the "Chair Man." At the flap opening sat the Fire Man. He would replenish the wood, spread the ashes, pick up the smoked offerings, and sweep the ground.

When all were seated, the chief opened his ceremonial bundle and removed the contents: an eagle-feather fan, a gourd rattle, tobacco and corn husks, a staff, and an eagle-bone whistle. In the center of the tipi was a fire with the logs placed in a "V." It flamed at its apex, which faced the Road Man.

In front of the Road Man was a three-inch-wide, six-foot-long crescent-shaped altar representing the moon, another traditional mother of humankind, made of wet sand. Its open ends faced the flap. After the Road Man blessed the symbolic items from his bundle, he placed his own special peyote cactus head, Chief Peyote or "Father Peyote," on top of the crescent altar on small branches of sage. Father Peyote was the focal point in the ceremony—it would keep us together on the road. It had been given to the chief by his grandfather. He told us to look at it, and it would teach us.

After his brief preamble, the Road Man had little to say. Each of us held the keys to our own path. The medicine would help us find our way to help the Road Man to assist us.

The Drum Man picked up his instrument. A rope and tiny round pebbles anchored the hide cover to a small, black, three-legged iron kettle half filled with water and chunks of charcoal. He drummed five or six beats a second. The drum music was strong, rhythmic, hypnotic, and I hummed with the beat.

We rolled the "opening smoke," placing sweet tobacco in corn husks. It had an anise-like taste and I coughed uncontrollably. Each smoker released a prayer with his or her smoke, and the whispy tendrils rose through the hole in the ceiling to the sky, taking the prayers to God. Fire Man carefully dragged some coals from the fire with a curved stick and piled them inside the crescent so that Cedar Man could sprinkle the cedar upon them as a fragrant accompaniment to the ascending prayers. All the participants blew and patted the smoke on to themselves. When we had completed this first smoke, we placed the butts on the edge of the altar for the Fire Man to pick up.

A bunch of fresh sage was passed from member to member, and each of us removed a few leaves to rub on our hands. Sage has traditionally been sacred to the Indian; the peyote people say it was the first plant God gave to the Earth Mother.

Then came the peyote—in a bowl, watered down into a loose cereal. (I have since eaten it as a dry powder, chewed it whole, or taken it as dried slices.) I gagged when I swallowed it—it was unbelievably bitter. Later I wanted to leave to vomit, but the Road Man told me it was okay to vomit right there.

Have you ever vomited in front of a group of strangers? It breaks down boundaries faster than anything I've yet discovered. No big deal. The Fire Man shovels and sweeps up the vomit. No one seems to notice, much less mind. The Road Man came to me and waved his fan over me as I inhaled deeply. He said it was supposed to come up, and here everything can be revealed without shame. I felt better.

The drum, gourd rattle, and staff were passed clockwise all night. We each had a chance to play them while singing if we chose to do so. In this ceremony, participants chant, smoke, and pray, and together create a catalyst for reflection. When worshipers finished their chants and songs, the Road Man sprinkled cedar onto the coals, and the sweet smoke rose animatedly from the fire.

After the first round of songs, Cedar Man smoked tobacco and prayed for healing for members of the circle who were absent because of illnesses. He asked a special blessing for the leaders of the nation, for the soldiers who serve it, for the sick and the poor, for rain, for crops, and for all the creatures of the earth. He beseeched Grandfather/Creator to bless the Native American Church, all its members, and all other people who want peace and brotherhood.

The singing continued. Participants took as much peyote as they felt was needed to guide them on their paths.

As the Road Man waved his fan at the cedar, I saw the black and white feathers melding into his flesh. His forearm became the wing of an eagle. I felt myself being waved upward along with the cedar smoke—I was rising out of my body. I became frightened for a moment that I might waft out through the top tipi hole. I was floating, looking at myself disembodied. I wanted to reach out to hold onto the chair, but I could not move my arm. I tried to speak, but no words came.

The Road Man saw my lips moving and the tears I did not even feel. He sprinkled water on my face and touched me, leaving his hand on me. "Look at the Father Peyote," he said. He refocused my attention and told me to stay with it.

The Road Man told me later that only the body is grounded. The spirit soars and tears speak. I have returned to that memory since. It has taught me how to feel small, to appreciate specialness in things ordinary, to be less serious about knowing.

An overwhelming sense of well-being came over me as I stared at the Father Peyote. The colors were incredibly vivid; the songs were unbelievably melodic; and the coals formed a sparkling, volcanic mosaic.

At midnight Fire Man passed around a pail of water and a cup after blessing them with special smoke and a prayer. All drank, and Drum Man poured water on his drum and shared some of it with the Earth Mother beneath his feet.

With the coming of dawn the night visions dissipated. The Road Man greeted the sun with his eagle-bone whistle and his morning song. "First Woman," who sits to the left of the Road Man, then got up and left the tipi. That night she was represented by the sponsoring family's maternal aunt, but sometimes she may be the Road Man's wife or a birthday child's mother. She returned with water, cornmeal, dried meat, and fruit. She blessed the food and water and prayed for the assembly. Without her prayers this night's ceremony would not be acceptable, as words spoken to the Creator without First Woman's light of dawn blessing would not be heard. This part of the ceremony sort of reverses the story of Eve, the fruit-bearing temptress who brought about Adam's fall. Here, civilization is sustained by women. At the same time, Fire Man fashioned the coals within the crescent into the form of the peyote bird, which carries the soul to God.

After our symbolic meal, the Road Man led the closing rite of prayers while he returned the peyote symbols to his case. The hide was removed from the iron kettle and the lumps of charcoal placed on the glowing coals of the fire. The water from the drum was poured along the upper edge of the crescent altar.

I stood to go outside. Except for a short break at about midnight I'd now been sitting for almost six hours straight and had no back pain.

Before leaving the tipi, people spoke of their appreciation for having been there. The Road Man gave his ceremonial bundle to the Fire Man, who carried it out, and we all emerged behind him, talking of the night's experience.

Moments of insight and new awareness—altered states of consciousness—can occur any time or anywhere. Usually we try to control the experience and minimize its potential impact by devising methods to cover it up or explain it, rather than appreciate or reexperience it.

My experience has been that if you feel it as real, go with it, and don't diminish it. Trust your unconscious; it will take you to a place of enlightenment. It is a part of you that usually guides you to a new place that offers nothing to fear. If you only see what seems to make you comfortable, then you are always destined to relive the old experiences and remain closed to discovering new levels of your own being.

In our culture, any experience of the intuitive, unencumbered, less controlled part of the mind has generally been repressed. Artists and others of creative mind know that the unconscious must be uninhibited to make the associations that produce new understanding. It is being open to the unconscious that allows insight to blossom into conscious comprehension.

Children are too often reprimanded for expressing their imagination, and soon they lose touch with it. In our culture the rational problem-solving part of our minds has become ascendant. But we must never lose sight of the intuitive, right-brain processes. Our obsession with what is rational is the most unfortunate consequence of a contemporary scientific attitude that reduces all "being" to a single dimension, to what can be seen, repeated, proven, and quantified by "objective" research and observation. Such dogmatism in the way we view reality limits our ability to open ourselves up to the multilevel states of being that may also have something to teach us.

Erich Fromm knew that our rational, scientific, production-and-consumption orientation closes us off from the other parts of our selves. Herbert knew that the mind is mysterious, and Santiago knew that to heal you must be able to dance, to hear the music from deep within. All knew that we are doomed if we don't follow the walk to our souls.

The Road Man says peyote is a messenger to one's soul. Now I want to tell you two stories about how Father Peyote spoke his message.

Chapter 6

 ## DELBERT AND BILLY: TWO PEYOTE STORIES

Delbert

When I learned that I had an appointment to see a man who had confessed to the murder of a baby, I felt repugnance even before I met him.

A psychiatrist's opinions, like anyone else's, may be colored by his or her preconceptions, but we hope that our professional training can reprogram us so we will not be forever bound by those preconceptions. I made a sincere effort to shelve my initial disgust and to read the patient's file and the police report. They did nothing to relieve my repugnance.

Delbert had a rap sheet listing dates, charges, and legal dispositions that had begun in 1959, when he was twenty. He had been arrested more than forty times, mostly for drunken and disorderly conduct. In 1962, following a guilty plea for a burglary offense, Delbert was committed to a California federal correctional facility, where he had served approximately three years. Since his release in 1965, he had lived in remote Navajoland with his wife and seven children ranging in age from ten years to fifteen months.

It was obvious from his dossier that Delbert's substantial drinking problem had not abated since his release from prison. The record showed numerous "drunk and disorderly" arrests on and off the reservation. A mechanic by trade, Delbert had been unemployed for five years and was receiving welfare.

For a week, from a Saturday to the next Sunday, Delbert had been in Holbrook, Arizona, occupying himself by drinking a cheap wine called Twister. On Sunday, his niece Sarah and her husband, Pete, found Delbert drunk and took him to their home in Holbrook for breakfast, then to her mother's home. En route, Delbert purchased another two-dollar bottle of Twister. He spent Sunday night in his sister's house with her five children, together with Pete and Sarah and their two children.

On Monday, while the older children were in school and the adults were gone, Delbert began to hear awful voices that threatened his life and refused to go away. That night, he was unable to sleep because of the maledictions.

The terrible voices faded on Tuesday but returned in the night. Unable to stand the sounds within his head, Delbert ran out of the house, tearing off his jacket and cap in an effort to hide from the voices. He was convinced that unseen presences wanted to kill him.

After running for an hour or more, Delbert became exhausted and returned to the house. He woke Pete and Sarah and asked them to take him to a nearby tribal police substation so that the officers could lock him up in the back of the police panel truck and allow him to go through his drunken "fits" without injuring himself or others.

The couple took Delbert to a police officer's home about 1 A.M. But the officer said he couldn't arrest Delbert or take him into custody because Delbert was not then intoxicated. Instead, at the officer's direction, they took Delbert to the community paramedic, who gave him two tranquilizer capsules and told him to go to bed.

The tranquilizers had no effect. Delbert was still hearing the voices and was a long way from sleep. He moaned that he was afraid of himself because of the voices. He convinced Pete and Sarah to tie him up with a lariat and with belts. After tying him up and locking him in a room by himself, Pete and Sarah and all the children went to bed.

From approximately 2 A.M. that morning until dawn, Delbert continued to hear the threatening voices. Some told him that he would be better off dead, because if he got loose he would kill all the children in the house. Others told him to go ahead and get loose, that he would not hurt anyone. Delbert began struggling to free himself of his bonds.

During the struggle he awoke Sarah and shouted for her to get help so he could be subdued and prevented from hurting someone. Twisting and loosening his bonds, Delbert warned Sarah that if he did get free, he was going to kill someone.

Pete and Sarah gathered all the children and fled the house in their pick-up truck. In their panic, however, they failed to take their five-month-old son, who was in a crib in the living room. Sarah jumped out of the truck and ran back into the house to get the baby. As she entered the house, she saw Delbert break through the locked door of his room and lurch into the living room with a knife in his hand. Then, in horror, she watched him decapitate her son.

Delbert bolted from the house, still brandishing the knife. He chased several members of the family and attacked another of his sister's daughters. During his rampage, he suddenly turned the knife on himself and stabbed himself in the throat. Unsuccessful in his effort at self-destruction, he threw the knife away and begged the police, who had by now arrived at the scene, to kill him so that he would not harm anyone else.

The Navajo police took Delbert to the Window Rock jail. During the ride, he continuously heard voices telling him he was going to die. Once the police learned he was hearing voices, they took Delbert to the hospital in Fort Defiance where he was given a tranquilizing injection.

Now, as Delbert awaited trial for killing the baby, the authorities of the district court in Flagstaff wanted me to offer an expert opinion as to whether he was capable of distinguishing whether his actions were right or wrong at the time of the crime. They also wanted me to assess whether or not Delbert could have controlled himself.

Two weeks later Delbert arrived in my office, accompanied by federal marshals. He had a chain belt around his waist to which his wrists were handcuffed. There were also chains around his ankles.

It was an interesting way to conduct an evaluation. After all, I am a psychiatrist. People are supposed to share with me their innermost selves, in the hope of gaining new insight and changing their lives. And, certainly, they are to come to me because they want to, not because they have to. Everything Delbert said to me, however, could be held against him. The atmosphere hardly promoted open sharing.

Being asked to decide whether someone is responsible for criminal conduct is a difficult problem for a psychiatrist. According to the enlightened Ninth Circuit Rule, if at the time of an offense a person's conduct was the result of a mental disease or defect that rendered the person unable to appreciate the wrongfulness of his or her conduct (including moral wrongfulness) or to be unable to conform his or her conduct to the requirement of law, then he or she is not guilty by reason of insanity. Intoxication can be the cause of a mental defect, but since people choose to drink, most juries find intoxication insufficient justification for a judgment of innocence. Psychiatrists have been empowered to render these decisions, even though we invariably disagree with one another.

I once attended a training seminar directed at psychiatrists who provided expert witness testimony. The week-long course featured Supreme Court justices, appellate court judges, district attorneys, police chiefs, and some jurors from the celebrated trial of Sirhan Sirhan, the man who assassinated Robert Kennedy in 1968.

The jurors talked about listening to expert testimony from several psychiatrists who had evaluated Sirhan. After hearing a number of conflicting reports, the jurors finally chose to discard all the expert opinions. They themselves decided that if Sirhan could have so meticulously planned the assassination—knowing where to park his car, where to stand for a clear shot, how to negotiate the escape route—he couldn't be all crazy. So much for the expert testimony.

In my office, Delbert was alert and aware of both his present surroundings and the events that had brought him to me. He presented no evidence of psychotic thinking, no conspicuous signs of craziness.

Delbert told me that he had been reared in a sheepherding family. His father drank chronically, as did his brothers and sisters. Delbert had attended boarding schools from the time he was eight because BIA social workers felt that his home environment was not conducive to a healthy upbringing. He went home only for summer vacations. Delbert didn't do well scholastically, but he was excellent with his hands. He wanted to become a mechanic, but such course work was not available in the curriculum at that time.

Delbert told me, with sadness, that from the time he was fifteen years old at boarding school he had drunk heavily. He had probably been a chronic alcoholic since that time, was expelled from school for drinking, and had not held a steady job since.

During the last five years, he had been mostly unemployed, spending his time drinking cheap wine. He binged weekly, with or without money. There were always friends to share a bottle with him.

He stayed away from his family during these times, sometimes for weeks, until somebody fetched him. He had been in delerium tremens at least three times. These terrifying alcoholic hallucinations made him paranoid. Sometimes he didn't get the full-blown hallucinations and terrors—more often just the shakes and some perceptual distortions. On the night at his sister's house, the terrors had taken complete control.

Delbert knew he had killed his niece's baby and felt terrible guilt about it, but he didn't believe that he had committed the murder. It was the alcohol that did it, that made him do it.

Many Indian alcoholics—and their communities—look at such behavior that way—the drinker is never held responsible for his or her behavior while drinking. The abuse of alcohol is perpetuated by this tacit understanding that a drinker can say or do things while drunk that would be impossible to express otherwise.

My first reaction to Delbert's story was to look for some reason to find him guilty of his unspeakable crime. But as I listened to Delbert relate his history, it became clear that he was suffering from an acute alcoholic hallucinosis during the horrible night at his sister's house. I concluded that he was suffering from a mental disorder that made it impossible for him either to appreciate the wrongfulness of his conduct or to be able to conform his behavior to the requirements of law. Because of his history, his loss of connection to a sustaining culture, his years of losing himself to liquor, he had done terrible harm.

He felt himself somewhere between guilty and innocent; he knew he did it, but it wasn't really he that did it. But the law doesn't provide such a category. There was a plea bargain. Delbert was convicted of the lesser charge of involuntary manslaughter, rather than first-degree murder. He would spend more than six years behind bars.

In prison, Delbert met another young Navajo who had been incarcerated for armed robbery. This young man was visited regularly by a Road Man from the Native American Church. Delbert listened to his friend. There were few other people with whom he communicated; in Arizona's prisons inmates tend to band together according to ethnic groups.

Delbert was alternately fascinated by and skeptical of the church. He had been aware of it on the reservation, but although as many as half the people he knew were members, he had never been a participant.

The Road Man was permitted to visit inmates, but not to conduct services. He could only talk about the church and its traditions and discuss its precepts with the Indian residents. Delbert told me that the Road Man was a spellbinding storyteller. Delbert learned that peyote had been given to the Navajos at the beginning of creation, but that his people had not then been ready to receive it. Because of the Navajos' lack of awareness, the gift had been given to the people of the south.

In his first year of imprisonment, Delbert spoke to the Road Man about his guilt and shame. He told him that he wanted to return to the reservation, yet he was also afraid to go back to face the people who knew what he had done.

The Road Man told Delbert that he could follow peyote's path and seek a new vision, a new meaning for himself. He said peyote was a good way and that its power was a blessing to share among friends. Delbert felt so drawn to the concept that he knew he would participate on his release.

Six and a half years later, the Road Man sponsored a meeting for Delbert. That first night Delbert looked into the fire and saw his lined face as shriveled and old. In the green-flamed coals he saw the remnants of broken wine bottles.

The Road Man saw Delbert gasp, and he went to him at once. He waved his eagle fan over him and told him to focus on the sacrament on the altar. It would provide the answer. And Delbert knew that it already had.

He became a regular participant in the Peyote Church. He has never had another drink.

Billy

Billy and I worked together when he served as a physician's assistant on an isolated Indian reservation. For years he had been overworked—the longevity of physicians in this place was measured in months, not years.

Billy was the only health professional within a hundred miles. People figured it was his job to be available, so he was always "on call." He asked for relief, but nobody else was available. He asked for a transfer, but no one wanted to change places with him.

With no other relief in sight, Billy started drinking more and more heavily. One day when the pressure became overwhelming, he barricaded himself inside his house. Armed with an impressive array of artillery, he challenged all comers to try to get him.

I got a call asking what to do. I said, "Don't get too close to the house!"

I didn't know Billy personally then; but after hearing what he was doing, it didn't take much insight to see that he wanted us to take him seriously. I told the authorities to get a friend to tell Billy that we heard him now, loud and clear. We would find another place for him if he came out without his weapons.

The offer worked. Billy entered an alcohol treatment program. After the thirty-day in-patient program, he was reassigned to another job with the proviso that he attend Alcoholics Anonymous meetings and that he see me.

Being sober was a new experience for Billy. An Eastern band Cherokee, he had been raised in North Carolina by his sister. He had been drinking regularly since he was ten. He enlisted in the Army and got married at seventeen. Following his first military tour of duty, he had organized a country-western band and played all over Europe. He played, partied, and drank heavily.

When the wear of that life-style finally got to him, he had reenlisted in the service. He had been trained as a medical technician, and subsequently he went on for specialist training. After twenty years with the military, Billy retired to enter the Indian Health Service. By this time, he had been divorced and remarried four times.

The service desperately needed physicians' assistants, especially in the most underserved, isolated Indian reservations. Billy had been ready, excited, committed, and he had worked his butt off.

To talk with Billy was to be seduced by a hypnotic drawl. He was a smooth-tongued, country-style raconteur. Billy told me that he lived in a brothel as a boy and regularly endured the taunts of other children. He got into fights with such frequency that the authorities prohibited him from going to school. Billy had learned to play the guitar on a cigar box contraption, and he could sing the blues and those strangely haunting, mountain-hollow laments.

Many people who come to see me really don't want to hear what I have to say. A therapist's best students are those who already believe that he has something to tell them, rather than those who have to be convinced.

Billy was ready to learn. He told me that he knew something about sadness, and he was ready to give it up. He wanted to learn how to avoid more sadness. Through his sessions with me and his involvement in A.A. meetings, he was freeing himself of the alcohol that had produced his broken marriages, his panic, his life of sadness.

At A.A., Billy's natural charm made him an immediate winner. Billy said that he could "let his lip rap flap faster than molasses on a baby's ass." In meetings, he was confronted with an assortment of accomplished people as well as the hustlers, the frightened, and the lonely, and he learned from their stories.

Billy became involved with a new Universalist church and also with a woman about thirty years younger than he. He was still whooping and hollering in the western bars and remembering his old rodeo days of hard drinking and "buckle bunnies," but now he was drinking 7-Up or Perrier. He sometimes missed the taste of good "sippin' whiskey," he said. I assured him that I was appreciating it for both of us.

He was finding his own way, celebrating first a week, then a month, and then a year off booze. His relationship with the young woman moved him away from his preoccupation with his three young daughters, who had moved to Alaska with his estranged wife. Billy told me that he now had more energy than he had had in the last ten years. In the middle of this frolicsome relationship, Billy came to the office one day complaining of some difficulty in swallowing and a hoarseness in his throat. He saw a specialist, who said it was a little irritation of the vocal cords.

But in two weeks it didn't get any better, and after an X-ray he was told that something was displacing his windpipe. It looked like a growth that might have spread from his right lung. Additional tests revealed a virulent, small-cell lung cancer that had spread throughout his neck. For me, this was the first time that, in the middle of a treatment relationship, my patient was found to have an inoperable tumor.

Billy was stunned, angry, and overwhelmed. He steadfastly told me that he was going to "kick the cancer's ass." Billy read the literature and understood the odds. There was almost no chance he would last five years; most people don't last a year. Billy got on with the business at hand, meeting the new challenge. He was placed on a chemotherapeutic program and lost his hair. He vomited day and night.

I visited him weekly—at home when he couldn't move or at his little clinic, where he had joined a cancer self-help group. It is always helpful to talk with people who walk the same walk.

Our meetings were even more passionate and intimate. When you're dying, there is nothing to lose by looking at the truth and no time to waste doing anything else. It's remarkable how much you can deal with in an atmosphere devoid of bullshit.

Billy bought wigs and had fun with the varied hair styles—curly-headed wigs and short-parted coiffures. He took them off for the kids in clinic who loved to feel his smooth dome. He told them he was an extraterrestrial visitor. They called him "B.P."

During this time, he told me that his father had died of cancer. Billy also remembered that his father had attended all-night Native American Church meetings. Knowing of my interest in traditional healing, Billy wondered if he could go to a Peyote Church meeting; we talked about it at length. Then I discussed it with a Road Man and arranged for the two of them to meet.

Billy read about the church with the same appetite with which he had studied his disease. He wanted to participate, and I sponsored a meeting for him. On the meeting night, the tipi was full. I was there with Billy and his girlfriend—not as his doctor, but as a sponsor and a fellow seeker.

The Road Man invited us to explain to the group why we had asked for the meeting. I shared the fact of Billy's cancer and what had already been done to treat it. I said that he had asked to participate in this service because it was the way of his father. Billy said he had come for their support, their prayers, and for the energy of the Spiritual Source.

After the opening songs were sung, we ate the medicine. Billy gagged. He was chronically nauseous anyway, and the bitter plant was excruciatingly difficult for him to swallow. The songs, the drumbeat, and the fire were trance-inducing. The medicine always works well when you come to it in truth.

At midnight, the meeting's focal point, Billy spoke. He said that he had never come to the Creator in this way before, but that he had also never been this needy before. Weeping, he told them of his wish to live, of old ways and new hope, and asked for God's help. He appreciated their being with him now.

When Billy had finished, the Road Man told Billy that this was a good way, and in the way of peyote we could all find knowledge to help us. He would do the best he could for Billy, but it was not he who did the work—he was only an instrument in the hands of the Creator. "I am the servant," he said. "The master is above. But I will pray and sing, and all of us here will join so that our voices can be heard."

The Road Man walked to the fire. Poking around in the ashes, he picked up a glowing coal the size of a peach pit and placed it on a metal jar lid. He walked back to his seat; then, taking the coal from the lid, he placed it in his mouth.

When you perceive things from an ordinary state of consciousness, you see only what you have already seen. It is hard to believe the new vision because it doesn't mesh with what you think you know. Many of us find it difficult to acknowledge any visionary experience because of this resistance to new ways of seeing. The visionary experience shakes old comfortable realities.

The Road Man saw the burning coal from some extraordinary consciousness as something that would not endanger him physically. The coal spoke to him. That particular coal reached out to him and said, "Take me. I am the one." Using his cheeks as bellows, the Road Man sucked in air until the coal was white hot—we could see it illuminating the inside of his mouth.

Then he leaned over and blew heat and sparks right onto Billy's neck and chest. Billy sat unflinching, transfixed in the magic. The Road Man took the coal out of his mouth, placed it back on the lid, and carried it back to the fire. Returning to his seat, he picked up his cedar bag.

Dipping his hand inside, he sprinkled cedar onto the coals. He told us that the cedar gave color and smell to our prayers. We could see our words and send them on the wings of his eagle fan to be lifted to the Spiritual Source. The eagle is the messenger; it can fly high and serve as an intermediary between us and the Creator. His eagle-feather peyote fan had been handed down to him and he beheld its feathers now as if they were immortal.

"The eagle has faith, and we can learn from it," he said. It mates for life and lays its eggs only once a year in a place so inaccessible that there is room only for the nest. The nest is exposed to freezing cold and high winds, yet in this perilous place the eagle lays down its most precious gift. Our prayers should be like the faith of eagles. They will be sent skyward on eagle wings, to touch the ear of God.

At daybreak, the participants told Billy that they hoped their prayers would be found acceptable. They had prayed in the best way they knew how, and they too appreciated being there with him. The Road Man gave Billy the sage bedding on which the Father Peyote lay on the altar. To me he gave the bag of cedar and told me to use it in my prayers. I wondered at that moment what it might be like to put cedar down in the synagogue on the Day of Atonement.

Emerging from the tipi, we had coffee and donuts. Later we ate a big meal. Billy was not tired. His girlfriend, who had sat by his side all night long, looked pale and drawn.

We talked in the shade. Billy asked me if I believed in God.

"Einstein was asked that question," I told Billy. "And he said that he believed that there was Something that explained the spiritual harmony of the universe. That makes a lot of sense to me."

The day after the meeting, while he was showering, Billy wiped a layer of dead, black skin from his neck and chest. He said that he felt stronger.

Over the next four months, he began losing weight. His time was getting shorter. The tumor had spread to his abdomen and he was in constant pain.

He wanted to see his children and his estranged wife, who now lived in Nevada, so he drove to Las Vegas to visit them. When his wife opened the door of the motel room, she involuntarily shrank back in horror. Billy, formerly a husky 200-pounder, now weighed 120 pounds and his face was cadaverous. The children called out, "Daddy," and he cried unashamedly.

He took care of final business, rewriting his will and visiting with his other children. Billy knew that I was planning to go on vacation in only a matter of weeks. He felt abandoned, but he told me that he knew I had to go. I too felt I was abandoning him.

The week prior to my anticipated departure, Billy was admitted to the hospital weighing less than 100 pounds. He was taking narcotics for pain constantly, and he lapsed into periodic confusion.

On the evening before I was to leave, I got a call from the family to come to the hospital. Billy had lapsed into coma. He appeared to be dying. Would I come over?

Should I go to the movies with friends as planned and then to the hospital? No! To the hospital now! On my way out of the house, I remembered the cedar and hurried back inside to retrieve the bag I had stored since Billy's Peyote Church meeting.

When I arrived at the hospital, Billy was unconscious, his breathing irregular. Around his bed stood a colleague from Nevada, one daughter, and his estranged wife. I sat by his head, held his hand, and told him that I had brought the cedar that had been given to me when we were together in the meeting. Did he remember the Road Man's instruction that I use it in my prayers? Now was the right time.

I repeated it as I understood it: the cedar smoke would carry him on his way to the spirit world. It would guide him on his journey like prayers to God's ear. Each of us around the bedside would add our prayers for him, which would accompany him with our love.

After closing the door to his room, I ignited the cedar in an abalone shell and brushed smoke on Billy, on myself, and on all around. I spoke some words and handed the shell to the next person. Each one brushed the smoke and spoke to Billy. His friend told him that he would remember him not as he saw him at this moment, but in boots and saddle, and that he would miss him. Billy's wife said that she would tell the children those things that would make them proud of him. His daughter brushed the smoke all over and said, "Good-bye, Daddy, I love you."

After all had spoken, I put the shell down. Then I turned to look at Billy and I saw that he had died.

Cedar is sacramental in many tribes, as is incense in Catholic and Jewish holy places. They have in common the holiness of smoke, the amorphous substance that wafts prayers to the source, to God.

We dramatically underutilize potential healing sacraments, whether they are rituals or objects that can mean something to us. The cedar that I burned at Billy's bedside brought together the people around him in a special way and enabled them to say words that otherwise might not have come.

I'm ready to perform sacraments with the door open now because I understand better that healing is also a spiritual process. Psychotherapists and doctors are priests invested with special power to persuade the spirit to heal. If belief helps a patient to find comfort, and if we believe we can help patients, then we must invoke the power of all healing sacraments to do so—to help the patient grow and heal, or even to accept losses and death.

Now, if a patient believes in ritual and sacraments, I put down cedar. I use feathers and herbs. It isn't that I have any magic; it's the rituals and their sacramental quality—they *are* healing.

Chapter 7

 JOLENE

The Mohave graveyard was a flat, stone-strewn field with few gravestones. In the old days there had been no grave markers at all. The human ashes, following cremation, were simply covered with dirt and left unmarked.

The end was the end; there was no engraved immortality. One returned to the earth, the eternal source, to become a part of it, to nurture those coming after. Previous lives, like the land, were a gift for unborn generations. Connections to the people who ended there and to the place itself could help avert disasters.

The Mohaves, a small tribe living around Parker, Arizona, are reluctant to talk to me of death and rebirth, not because I am unsympathetic, but because I am not Mohave. The few rituals that remain to them are carefully handed down to other Mohaves as an oral tradition.

In general terms, the Mohaves see dying as just another aspect of the life cycle. As in the creation myths of most religions, death and rebirth are part of an unending circle that connects all Mohaves with those who came before and, ultimately, to their supernatural ancestors, Matavilya and Mastamho, who created the Colorado River, produced light, shaped the land, and separated the Mohave people into clans.

I have also come to interpret death as the final adaptation to life. Death is when the body parts no longer communicate with one another in the old language. Death is an expression of what we once knew as life, but in another form. The task of healing, as I see it, is to maintain communication within the body as long as it is sensible to do so.

The Mohaves believe that when one dies the spirit is freed and goes on a voyage to the spirit world to be reunited with all its ancestors, a passage the living are not to interfere with. The body is only a container for the spirit, a reminder of this earthly life. If the body is not cremated, it becomes a burdensome connection to the earthworld and makes the spirit voyage more difficult.

Thus, when someone dies, friends and relatives return all of his or her possessions or attachments to earth. Toys, photographs, special gifts, clothing—all are burned. The deceased's name is not mentioned anymore. After the Mohave cryhouse ritual, tears are no longer shed for the lost loved one. Tears weigh the spirit down and make the voyage difficult.

I first met Jolene when she was ten. Her mother, Gail, a light-complexioned Anglo, and her father, Gabe, a full-blooded Mohave, were friends of mine. Jolene was a tall, bright child, an honor student who attended college on a scholarship. She was elected one of sixteen official representatives (the youngest of them) of the state of Oregon to the National Women's Conference in Houston, Texas, in 1977.

Jolene was usually active and striving, but while away at school she became depressed. She wrote to her father, who in turn explained in a letter that the forces of evil could sometimes capture one's energies. Jolene said that she wanted to take a break from all work and school and no play. She wanted to reevaluate and rededicate herself. She told her father that she wished to come home at semester break. She felt burdened, and she had dreams of dying.

Gabe knew of the unconscious, of self-doubt, uncertainty, guilt, and pain. He agreed that his daughter should return to recharge her personal energy.

At semester break, however, Jolene decided not to come home. Gabe told her to go and sweat—he would send her the sage and herbs to do it in the traditional way.

Ritual cleansing has been a part of almost all cultures. Christians have baptism and sprinkling; Jews ritually immerse themselves before Yom Kippur, the Day of Atonement. Indians go to the sweat lodge to cleanse the body and the soul before ceremonial occasions. To speak and listen to the Creative Source in the sacred grounds, you must get yourself in the appropriate frame of mind and be as cleansed and new as possible.

Cleansing is another ritual that has lost its sacramental quality for us. Now we go to a health spa and sit in the sauna or steam room as a social event or a beautification scheme. The native tradition, however, teaches that the steam is the breath of our grandparents and that the rocks producing the steam are invested with the spirits of all the people who have gone before. Sweating, with your ancestors breathing on you, has a healing influence.

We need to learn to separate the ordinary from the sacred, to learn to appreciate the mystery in small things whose origins we forget. Steam, incense, and smoke and ritual paraphernalia like candles and fire remind us of those mysteries.

Gabe wanted Jolene to go into a steam room and see it in a cleansing way. Then she would be prepared to receive the spirit.

She could receive her message by dreaming, her father advised her, and she should use the dream message to overcome the dark influences and help restore her balance. She had to do it now, while she was vulnerable to the forces of darkness. To let it go longer would only make it harder to shake later. He compared the dilemma to a hardening jello mold: you could not ignore the forces of darkness, or they would harden you. They had to be exorcised—met and conquered. (I think it not a bad definition of neurosis: the forces of darkness capturing and holding you until your "jello" hardens.)

He told Jolene that he and other friends would pray for her. My friend believed that prayers in any form, songs, and silence were acceptable to God as long as they were sincere. And he told Jolene that she must pray too. Her healing must ultimately come through her own being.

Jolene took the herbs to a steam room and cleansed herself as her father had suggested. She did better in school and was no longer worried; she became more involved in campus activities. The dreams of death dissipated, but she later wrote to her father asking that she be cremated in the Mohave way if she died.

Before the school year was over, Jolene was riding in a small car with some friends. The car collided head-on with another and Jolene sustained a massive head injury. The doctor initially said that she would not survive. My friend went to the Midwestern medical center to be with his daughter.

Jolene was in a neurology intensive-care unit, a fantasyland of life-sustaining mechanical wonders that overwhelmed

Gabe. She was unresponsive, but he sat at her bedside and spoke to her.

There was no way to explain why the accident had occurred to his daughter, no way to determine why it should be Jolene lying there in a comatose state. As we had often said to one another, "shit happens."

Gabe was a father maintaining a connection with his daughter even though she was unconscious. He was speaking with her as she existed between worlds and helping her to make a choice between those worlds.

In the old way, he perceived Jolene as existing in another dimension of life. She could see and hear things that he could not, but he could remind her of life in this dimension by telling her of his thoughts and visions. He spoke to Jolene of their home and his wish to take her back with him. He described the desert sage and ocotillo, the river and the sacred mountains of the reservations on which they had lived. He talked about Tempe, the house they lived in while he attended graduate school. He talked about her sisters, her mother, himself. He told her that in the place where she now existed she could still hear him and that he would stay with her.

Six weeks after the accident, Jolene was medically stabilized and, still unconscious, was transferred to Phoenix. When I saw her, she did not appear to hear me. Gabe assured me that she did hear, for he had seen her move her eyes. By the seventh week, Jolene opened her eyes. Gradually she improved, at first responding to words by blinking her eyes. Later she pointed to printed cards to indicate when she wanted the television channels changed and other simple requests. She still could not speak or move.

One evening I asked Jolene if she remembered the events following the accident. By pointing to the cards, she picked out her recollections. She did not recall the intensive care unit at all—she remembered hearing, seeing, and smelling her Arizona home.

Some weeks later, Jolene developed respiratory problems, and she was placed on a positive pressure breathing machine and fed through a tube threaded into her stomach. She occasionally appeared in respiratory distress, but her spirits were good.

Eleven weeks following the accident, she could sit up strapped in a chair. Jolene remembered more and more of the time before and after the accident, but not of the accident itself. She recalled visions of her family, her favorite haunts, the swimming holes.

During this time she developed a complication from the tracheotomy tube in her neck. A stricture had developed at the place where the tube ended in her trachea, but it was not seen as a serious problem. Periodically Jolene became racked with fever. She developed pressure sores on her buttocks. Her lungs became clogged with infection, but she was alert.

One evening Jolene tapped her head and pointed toward the wall at her feet. Her father changed the direction in which she was lying, moving her so that her head pointed to the north. The Mohave cremate their dead with the head pointed south. Jolene was not yet ready to die.

One day, Jolene was found in bed with the tracheotomy tube expelled. The doctors manually held open the hole in her neck as they attempted to insert another tube, but it could not get beyond the narrowed opening. A smaller tracheal tube was tried. Jolene did not complain, but she winced in pain at the manipulation.

While the doctors prepared the operating room for surgical reinsertion of the tube, Jolene suffered cardiac arrest. Three hours after the tube had been found expelled, all resuscitation efforts had failed and Jolene was pronounced dead.

She was taken back to Parker, where her family would translate her body the old way—after an elaborate ceremony. Jolene would be cremated.

For two nights before the cremation, members of the Mohave community gathered in the cryhouse, a white building that adjoined the cemetery. Jolene's casket rested on a raised central platform; the mourners placed mementos of Jolene next to her body, and one by one they stood and spoke of her.

The witnesses spoke only of the good things about Jolene. Whatever the bad, such shortcomings are only the baggage of an earthbound existence and should be left here, they said. The dead should only be remembered for their goodness, thus freeing them to rediscover their ancestors in spiritual harmony. Gabe stood and said that it was fitting for Jolene to be cremated in the old way, because it was a reaffirmation of the rightness of that way, an expression of life that could not be improved upon, an ethic about life that remained undiminished with time.

The cryhouse was filled with tears. The rhythmic chanting and soft moans in the background helped me remember the Jolene I once knew on camping trips in the pines, in Earth's peaceful tipi. I felt a giant ball well up in my throat, but stopped it there. It has always been hard for me to let go of tears; I still struggle to accept that part of my truth, that soft, vulnerable part that smacks of childishness or weakness or lack of control.

Relatives from the Quechan, the Cocopah, and the Maricopas came to share in the ritual. Gail performed the mother's ritual task of removing her daughter's shoes, a part of the tribal ritual she found comforting in her loss.

For everyone there, the cryhouse and cremation reaffirmed their way. Each person knew that he or she too would end in that place; and there is some comfort, I think, in being able to grow accustomed in life to the place of one's death. Death rituals are a useful reminder of our own mortality: your time here is limited; we must do whatever has to be done now. They also allow people to connect with the spirit and remind us that everyone comes and goes from this earth.

Such recognition and acceptance of mortality seem lost in contemporary life. One of the failures of current psychological movements lies in their inability to acknowledge that one day there will be an end to becoming.

As dawn approached, the pallbearers, friends, and relatives all stood as the casket bearers lifted the coffin from the platform. The singers led us all in the procession outside. When we had all emerged, the singers stopped to turn eastward and greet the rising sun. We moved again, accompanied by the chants and rattles. Then we stopped to face north, then twice more to face west and south. The stops would remind Jolene of the directions she had experienced in life and would tell the spirit world that she would again touch those directions on her spiritual voyage.

At the burial site the bearers removed Jolene from the casket and placed her in a pit lined with logs, a funeral pyre was about seven feet long and four feet wide resembling a truncated pyramid. The chanters stood only ten feet away, facing the brilliant rising sun. The rest of us, at a distance of perhaps thirty feet, formed a circle around the pyre.

From a large foot locker the assistants removed blankets, unfolding and draping about thirty of them one by one over the log pile to protect Jolene on her journey. Their bright rainbow colors were the colors of life, I was told.

Then, from inside the trunk, came old toys and dolls that had been returned to her in the cryhouse. These too were stuck into the pile.

Friends and relatives chose to keep only a few reminders, bringing the majority of Jolene's possessions to the pyre, so that Jolene would be completely released from this world to embark on her voyage. The Mohave concept of ownership eliminates wills, probates, and recriminations.

The chants became more intense. Our people circle swayed. In the early morning light, the draped pyre was wrapped many times around with a ribbon of bright scarves. The assistants moved back, as the one who bore the fire torch lighted each corner of the pyre.

A woman standing beside me in the circle removed her loose-fitting blouse and dress. Others followed suit and walked slowly to the growing fire to throw their clothes into the flames. In the old days, they would have cut their hair and stripped naked.

When they rejoined the circle, we rhythmically began a side-stepping movement around the leaping flames, circling in time to the chanting. The heat became intense and the circle moved back. The chanters came closer and threw their rattles into the flames. All of earth life relating to Jolene would be consumed.

The flames now reached twenty feet in the air, and the sky rained fragments of embered cloth like an anointing powder. I shuddered at the feeling of her presence on me.

We danced until the flames subsided. Then the circle divided. One half moved clockwise, the other counterclockwise; and each participant shook the hand of every other, then moved to the benches to shake the hands of seated family members. Shortly, Gail and Gabe removed themselves from the scene and then, quietly, all the others left. The crying was over. After the funeral noise, the silence was eerie.

The fire would burn and smolder all day and night. The logs, tilted inward, would eventually collapse, and the ashes would fill the hole. By morning, only a thin layer of earth would be needed to cover the pit.

Jolene's spirit journey had begun, and the magical intaglios that had been carved centuries ago at the bases of sacred mountains in the Colorado River Valley would show her the way.

After the cremation, I sat with Gabe and Gail for a while at their house. Gabe said, simply, that Jolene had completed her circle here. Hers had been only a moment in an unending spiral. All Indian life symbols are circular, without beginning or end. Gail said that her daughter was now released to choose again what to be.

All rituals, all sacraments are ways of preparing us for the inevitable truth that disasters occur, that "shit happens." Most of them are small when compared to dying, but one day we too will make our journey into another space.

If I, as a physician, cure someone and aid him or her to become less vulnerable to that disease again, then I am a good doctor. But if I, as a doctor, cure someone, aid him or her to become less vulnerable to that disease, *and* help him or her to understand their place in the universe, then I am a healer.

All the great dancing healers I have met have enabled their people to build bridges over the unknowable gaps, the mysteries, of our existence. They deal directly with the transition of death, and they participate in ritualized mourning. Then they get back to the business of living.

Chapter 8

SAM OLD DOG AND HECTOR: TWO OUTSIDERS

Sam Old Dog

Modern society, as Erich Fromm tells us, has many unhappy, isolated prisoners. In this context, I think often of Sam Old Dog, a twenty-eight-year-old Sioux Indian who had been referred to me by the tribal court as a wife-beater.

Sam had been a radio man with a Special Forces unit in Vietnam. After the war, when he was living in Phoenix, sometimes little things would trigger a feeling of being overwhelmed by aspects of his environment beyond his control, and rages would come suddenly upon him. On other occasions, he would sit silently and stare at nothing. Sometimes he drank to forget his misery and bewilderment.

His wife had become more than a little concerned that his erratic behavior would one day produce more than a beating for her. She feared that he might shoot her.

Sam was worried too. He felt bad about the beatings, and he told me that he had also taken to stalking road signs at night. He would sneak up on highway markers and obliterate them with a high-powered rifle that he kept hidden underground.

Sam Old Dog came into the world as a result of an out-of-wedlock pregnancy. His mother quickly bequeathed him to her parents, and they moved to Los Angeles when he was less than two years old. He grew up in the shadow of the Los Angeles Coliseum, the only Indian in a predominantly black and Mexican-American neighborhood. Sam soon realized that he was *the* minority in a minority neighborhood, so he was never certain on whom he might rely in an emergency. He learned to cater to both the blacks and the Chicanos by becoming a comedian. As a "crazy Indian kid" he came and went as no one's enemy.

Sam Old Dog's grandparents were quite religious, and he went to church with them on Sundays. When he was fourteen his mother remarried, and she took Sam back after his enfeebled grandmother was institutionalized.

Sam did not get along well with his stepfather. He spent most of his time on the streets with friends and became part of the California 1960s scene. He smoked lots of marijuana, experimented with hallucinogens, and played volleyball on the beach. Only once did he have a "bad trip." At an outdoor concert the popular LSD guru Timothy Leary was dropping rose petals from a helicopter. The swirling sawdust kicked up by the whirling rotors settled on Sam's skin, and he hallucinated that he was being eaten by bugs.

In the midst of this bliss, he received a draft notice.

Sam found a friend who had also received his "greetings" from the local draft board, and together they decided to leave the country. Setting out in a psychedelically painted VW bus, the two protestors planned to sell dope along the way to Canada to cover expenses. By the time they got to Seattle, Sam Old Dog couldn't stand the grayness, the cold, the wind of the Northwest, and he decided to return home despite the draft and the Vietnam War. By the time Sam arrived back in California, his second induction notice had arrived. It included the promise that if he did not report this time, a warrant would be issued for his arrest. Sam reported for duty.

To Sam's surprise, he liked the army. He loved the camaraderie of basic training and marveled at how skillfully the military changed men. First the haircuts, then the uniforms; everyone looked the same and had the same purpose. He also remembered Audie Murphy, World War II's most decorated soldier. He fantasized returning as a hero to parades and a nation's grateful applause. Sam was a good soldier. He now drank beer and smoked dope only occasionally.

After basic training he was sent to a front-line battalion in Vietnam where he spent eleven months surrendering and recapturing the same hill. His entire tour was spent securing its perimeter. This cyclical effort of capturing and losing the hill nine times took the lives of 60 percent of the comrades with whom he had arrived in Vietnam.

Sam described to me his recollections of sitting on the mountain at night when the perimeter lights went out, knowing that he was in enemy country, that he could die. For every day he fought, Sam got a day off. If he fought longer, he received more time off. On those days off, when he came back to base, he disappeared with friends—first to drink, then to smoke opium-laced marijuana, and finally to shoot heroin. Finding a woman became secondary. Drugs dominated army life, he said. Officers were doing dope just like the enlisted men. The stuff was sold openly out of duffle bags.

He was twice detoxified from heroin. The first time Sam admitted himself to the base hospital because he thought he had malaria. The second time the habit was heavier and the withdrawal more painful; he kicked it alone while on patrol on the mountain, gulping down great quantities of Valium to help with the shakes and the terrible feelings of desperation.

Three weeks after this withdrawal, Sam was involved in an action on a village. As he advanced on foot, air support dropped napalm. He saw a little girl run out of a flame-engulfed hut. She was on fire, so he took off his radio pack and ran toward her, but she was dead by the time he got to her. He stood staring, then dropped his weapon and walked back to camp. When the medics examined him, he was mumbling.

From the base hospital Sam Old Dog was sent to an area receiving hospital. He was psychiatrically discharged from the service as a chemical "brain-fry," a casualty of drugs, not combat.

Sam returned to the streets of Los Angeles. Though he had done his job in the army, there were no welcome-home parades, hardly even a hello. There were no jobs for soldiers who knew how to secure a hill in guerrilla country. Sam found himself unable to make new friends, and he lost touch with the old ones. He didn't belong anywhere.

He became seriously alcoholic. For a living he panhandled. Drunk or sober, he was still in Vietnam. When a Los Angeles traffic-watch helicopter flew over, Sam would sometimes scream and flee for cover under a parked car. On steamy summer afternoons, Sam could still smell the jungle.

At a bar, Sam met another Nam veteran who introduced him to the antiwar movement. He convinced Sam Old Dog that the only way his experience would make sense was to tell it to others who understood. Old Dog went with him to a meeting and became marginally involved with the group. It was not really his thing. He remained detached from women and continued to drink heavily.

Finally, after an arrest, the judge told him it was either jail or a treatment program. Old Dog picked an alcohol treatment program for Indians in Arizona. He was amazed to discover that the other residents looked to him as a leader. Indian country turned out to be one of the few places where being a Vietnam veteran was an honor. Returning warriors who had defended their land always received respect.

In the program, Sam also found a woman who helped him open up to loving, and they got married. Their relationship was good but sometimes Old Dog still had the dreams of the war, even ten years after his discharge. An added complication arose when he wanted his wife to get pregnant, and she couldn't. Sam blamed her; he blamed himself; he blamed the war.

When I first saw him, my barely suppressed feelings about the basic immorality of war kept me from being truly receptive to him and his war stories. After listening to him, I knew that I had confused my attitude about the warrior with my feelings about the war. I had avoided looking at Vietnam that way for a long time.

We talked about helplessness, fear, and rage, but it was not in my office that Sam got turned around. He anchored his center in his roots as an Indian and his pride as soldier, and he found those anchors through ritual.

Sam joined an Indian veterans group that participated in Gourd Dances, social events that are opened by a procession of modern-day warriors bearing the colors. Decked in traditional blankets, they affix their armed services medals to these uniforms. Singers around the great drum chant songs honoring warriors as they enter.

Before each occasion, the warriors prepare themselves by sweating. Old Dog described his first experience in the sweat lodge to me:

Twelve men sat close together in a small, canvas-covered igloo of willow branches. In the center was an earth pit in which hot stones were placed. The ceremonial leader lit a corn husk cigarette and passed it around and the men washed themselves in the smoke. The leader sprinkled water and cedar on the coals, and spoke to the rising steam:

> With this breath of the rock people, we will heal the pains in our bodies and our minds. This way has sustained our elders and it will sustain us. This way takes care of the winged creatures and those that crawl upon the Earth, those that walk or swim, and all that grows upon the Mother Earth. Treat all with respect, and treat yourself with respect. Our skin is the color of the Earth Mother; we are of her, and she is of us. If we remember these things, they will keep us together. Let us walk tonight with pride. We are warriors who carry the spirit of those who went before.

The leader then dipped the sage wand into the bucket in front of him and sprinkled all the participants. In the darkness Sam cried. The leader added cedar to the stones and the men bathed themselves in the sweet smell. They went in and out of the lodge four times. During each round, another member led the prayer.

When it was Sam's turn to lead, he said that he had never prayed this way before, that he didn't know how to do it, but that he wanted to say a few words in the best way he knew

how. The others encouraged him. Sam said that he was overcome with ugliness sometimes and that he was ashamed for
what he had done to his wife and to himself. The others mum-
bled their understanding and encouragement. Many had
been there too.

Old Dog kept going to sweats and to Gourd Dances. He
stopped beating his wife.

All sacraments offer healing.

Hector

Regardless of all the warnings in the psychoanalytic literature about self-disclosure, I now freely tell stories about
myself. I tell my patients Hasidic tales and Indian stories; I
sing songs and even make revelations about my own pain and
personal struggles. Of course, I choose very carefully those
stories that I share, but storytelling is important to my patients.
It is what psychiatry is about; you listen to people tell their
stories, and you tell yours.

The Indian worldview is pragmatic—you can't know anything until you've done it; anything else is a guess. If my
Indian patients are going to believe I can help them, it will
be because I've told them about the things that I have done,
not just the things that I know. This knowledge from experience is why you have to be gray to be able to heal.

The stories show that each person must become one with
the truth of his or her head, lips, and heart. If you say what
you really mean and you believe what you say, then you stay
healthy.

This is Hector's story.

From the time of creation, says Pima history, the Arizona
desert had rivers. Today there are only parched cracks in the

earth. The once-flowing waters lie entrapped in dammed lakes, serving the thirst of new desert cities. The Hohokam, the ancient ancestors, once dug canals by hand to trap the sudden downpours, so the precious rain could be used to grow food. Now rain water gets sucked into the dry earth within moments, or it floods the land because the river can no longer hold it.

In the old days the Pima were mainly farmers, becoming warriors only to resist their nomadic, hostile neighbors. Today they still live on their ancestral lands, but without much water. The culture and politics of the Southwest center around water. Whoever gets it thrives. Arizona's tribes are not doing well in this war either. They consistently lose to the cities, the mines, and the corporate farmers.

Hector's mother left the Pima reservation for Phoenix. Her first husband had disappeared in an alcoholic fog. The land could not sustain her, so she would try the city. But she could not support her children and her own alcoholism too.

When he was two years old, Hector was left with a blind grandmother back on the reservation. Three other siblings went elsewhere. Each day he looked at this gentle woman, with those clouded globes in her corroded sockets, and he loved her. She held him closely, and he guided her steps and picked up twigs whose bark she would strip with her teeth to make the baskets for which she was famous. "A blind basketweaver," marveled tourists.

Hector learned to weave too, while listening to her stories. They slept in the same room, on one bed. When he got older, he made the evening fire, tilting the sticks vertically to burn more slowly. He would later say that he had never known such peace.

When Hector was eleven years old, his grandmother died from the complications of long-standing diabetes, an illness that plagues the Pimas. Hector cried then, but he has not for a long time since. His grandmother buried, Hector went back to Phoenix with his mother. His grandmother had never let Hector return to his mother, out of her love for him, for she knew that her daughter was still drinking.

After Hector moved into his mother's house, he began some peculiar behaviors. He would stalk neighborhood cats and lock them up in a discarded refrigerator. After they had suffocated, he would hold elaborate funeral services. His teacher sent home a copy of an essay that Hector had written describing the evisceration of a baby prior to its burial. At this teacher's suggestion, his mother brought him to see me. Together we talked about death and dying and grandmothers and departures, and he seemed to improve.

After a year I lost track of Hector. But as a freshman in high school he reappeared when his counselor wrote to me asking for his records. Hector had been placed in a learning disabilities program because of his marginal academic performance, and the teaching staff wondered about his psychological status. Soon they sent Hector back to me.

The teenage Hector was nicely dressed and spoke well. He laughed about old dead cats; they were just a bad memory. He had friends of all kinds and was well accepted.

Then why wasn't he doing well in school? "Because of a lot of stuff at home." His mother was chronically alcoholic; among his brothers, one was a transvestite, one was retarded, and another was in the penitentiary. There was not a lot of love and no real home for him there. Hector wanted refuge, but I told him that it was all but impossible to find shelter for a minor who is neither flagrantly crazy, criminal, nor a runaway.

A month later he encountered the last straw when his family taunted him about his new girlfriend. He had fallen in love with a waitress and left her big tips. She appeared interested in him and promised to meet him outside the restaurant. He took his money out of the bank and continued to tip her well. His family found out and mocked him: "That white girl's just using you for a dumb Indian." Hector cursed at them and walked out, vowing never to return.

I still couldn't find a place for him. There was nowhere for Hector to go.

One week later he appeared in the emergency room accompanied by the police. They had found him wandering the streets, carrying a shopping bag and wearing nothing. In the bag was a pair of sneakers with which Hector said he would lead the American forces against the encroaching Communist invaders. The bag also contained a transistor radio, with which Hector picked up the enemy broadcasts and transmitted coded messages. Now I could hospitalize him.

In his dreams Hector reported being devoured by giant, sightless dinosaurs, only to find that he could live safely in their stomachs. He would live forever, he was convinced, because dinosaurs only eat vegetables. He became a vegetarian.

I told him that the giant reptile represented his blind grandmother. He wanted her to take care of him again. He wanted out of his world and back into her nest.

But direct interpretations, however insightful, rarely change behavior. I don't use them anymore, because people can find more ways not to hear them than you have ways of saying them.

In the hospital, Hector participated in a psychodrama where people act out what's on their minds within a group of people who can give input and discuss the individual's pain. A boy in the group talked about his prostitute mother; he wished that he had never been born. The group translated his fantasy into a whole production number and created a new birth for him: he could pick his ideal mother and be reborn.

While someone was pulling the boy out of a vaginal tunnel made of sofa cushions, Hector suddenly jumped in to grasp his arms and shouted, "Don't be stupid. Stay inside or they'll eat you!"

The group leader asked the entrapped boy which way he wanted to go. Others in the group could help him if he chose to come out, but only he could make such a decision. The kid decided to come out.

The others pulled his legs to help him emerge into the world. But Hector resisted, tugging at the boy's arms, crying, and screaming, "No! No! There is nothing out there!" When the others prevailed and the boy was "born," Hector banged on the cushions, cursing with rage at the group's stupidity. It was a real breakthrough for the boy, and it happened without interpretation or explanation of why he felt as he did.

Later, Hector acted out his own rebirth with the group. At the crucial moment he decided that he too wanted to come out. With that decision, he improved rapidly. Once Hector decided to emerge from the protective womb of his past, he released a lot of negative feelings—primarily his rage at his mother, and at his grandmother for dying. His medication was eventually stopped.

Hector told me that when he was a child he had been treated by a medicine man. He remembered that the healer had sung and blown on him. He wanted to see a medicine man again, so his relatives found one for him. I wanted to meet the man and go to the ceremony too.

Can one cure by breath and smoke? I had been taught to think seriously about even touching a person goodbye, much less sucking or blowing on someone. But I wanted to learn.

The medicine man, Francisco, was an old man—how old he didn't know. Francisco knew Hector's childhood story, and I filled in details about his recent experiences. The old man thought Hector had an insufficient life force to sustain him. His life force had been compromised, maybe even before his birth. His mother may have violated a taboo, perhaps touched some dead animal. She had separated her life from Hector while he was yet in the womb. (Alcohol can do that.)

From the Pima perspective, everything has potential power because everything is invested with energy—not only people, but animals, plants (especially mushrooms, cactus, corn, and tobacco), and even stones, from small rocks carried on one's person for their protective power, to large craters, canyons, volcanoes, or earthquakes—all are expressions of the potential energy of the universe.

Francisco thought that he could strengthen Hector's life force by removing some illness-producing remnant within him. I used to think this kind of stuff was self-deception, pure and simple, because my training emphasized that behavior was the result of processes inside your own mind. The thought of some kind of diabolical possession as a result of touching dead meat was just unbelievable. But I know that a lot of symptomatic illnesses are expressions of the violation of some taboo.

This concept of possession, whether by witchcraft or unconscious conflict, is what psychotherapy is about. All healers, including psychiatrists, strengthen people's life force by helping to remove destructive debris; some healers call it exorcising devils. I've discovered that this kind of healing always works better when you use more than words.

Pima curing ceremonies are normally performed at night. Although I work almost exclusively in the daytime, I know that in the darkness we can more clearly see the illusions, distortions, and ghosts that live in the imagination. I have found that holding groups at night, outdoors with a fire if possible, powerfully facilitates their purpose.

This ceremony was to be both a diagnostic and a curing session for Hector. Francisco and his helpers came together early to create the strength necessary to heal. They smoked the house with sage. The atmosphere was as if they were preparing for a struggle.

Francisco would "illuminate" Hector's belly by the use of feathers and fetishes and smoke so he could see the offending source. Once he could see the problem, he would be able to mobilize the specific positive strength necessary to counteract it.

Francisco and his associates approached Hector with chanting, singing, and the shaking of rattles. They blew smoke on him, sometimes bending only inches above him. Some blew smoke toward the chimney hole, seeking to push their completed songs and prayers toward the spirit world. Francisco smoked special tobacco and blew it on Hector, then retreated to the furthest corner of the house and waved an eagle-feather fan at the songs as they emerged from his mouth. He directed the songs at Hector and far beyond him.

Francisco rubbed earth and ashes around Hector's belly button. He waved the eagle fan over the boy and leaned over him. From Hector's belly button he sucked out some teeth. The medicine man showed the glistening, jagged pearls to Hector, and then the teeth disappeared.

When the ritual was over, Francisco and the others pressed their hands on Hector. During the next several days, they monitored him to see if the removal of the negative forces and the induction of positive ones would take hold.

None of this seems silly to me anymore. Francisco and I both perceived Hector's problem as one of maternal deprivation. I talked to Hector about his pain. Francisco removed the internal conflict more actively, just as the psychodrama group had forced Hector's commitment to life. All the methods worked together to help Hector in his healing process. He had been reborn, this time into health and life, and he could proceed without his old fears.

This is how I understand Hector's story. When it comes to understanding the mind, we are like children. Even if we someday know the brain and its chemistry, the mind will always have a mind of its own. The mind is a multifaceted jewel that snatches at whatever light comes in from many angles and creates a myriad of hues and colors. There are as many ways to see the light as there are ways to create it.

Chapter 9

TWIN BOY AND THE TOMATO LADY: TWO TALES OF WITCHCRAFT

Twin Boy

I was conducting a seminar about human behavior for personnel at an Apache reservation hospital when someone raised the issue of witchcraft. Did I really believe, I was asked, that someone could make another person ill by casting a spell?

Most questions are really statements in disguise. There is power in everything, I say, as I have come to understand it. Objects and animals as well as people can influence human behavior. And witches can devise ways to influence your spirit. Witchcraft is just another attempt to explain things, a way of dealing with the dark forces that appear to have influence over our lives. I had come to believe that many things and many people could make us ill, because we are all needy, vulnerable, and to some degree, suggestible human beings.

Indian traditions have a strong belief in spirits and the healing presence of sacramental objects. Witchcraft is just the opposite side of that view; it explains the concept of evil. A concept of evil is necessary to give us a sense of right and wrong, a way of knowing how to treat others. It is the way a society survives. We all know that people can do things to hurt us. We may call them evil, despots, inquisitors, or enemies; sometimes we call them witches.

When you believe in witchcraft you also believe that you can get rid of the evil spirit. The task is to find a power greater than that of the witch; it may be a totemic animal, a psychic, a medicine man, a ceremony, surgery, or the confessional.

Curiously, I cannot always determine the sole symptomatic cause of an illness, so I really can't say that it hasn't been caused by a spell. But I do have a way to remove "curses" that have been set in motion by pain and fear. Furthermore, I told the group, I have discovered that I can remove a curse better by doing something to it than by interpreting it.

The process of psychotherapy is, in a sense, a kind of witchcraft made complicated. The therapist removes "spells" by assisting the patient to discover a power within him- or herself that is greater than the power that produced the symptom.

If I'm working with someone who believes in a system of good and evil powers, then I help him or her find the power that's greater than the evil one. If the patient gives me clues to ways of finding that power by using certain words or revealing certain beliefs, then I can use that context to help the patient win the struggle. It's what Milton Erickson meant when he taught that the symbols must have meaning for the patient.

After my presentation, a woman named Marti asked to speak with me for a moment. Could I keep a secret? She wanted to tell me something that nobody else knew. I felt her urgency and assured her that whatever she wanted to say would be just between us.

Marti began by saying that she had become increasingly depressed over the past two years. Night terrors would awaken her and she couldn't fall back asleep. What was worse, she believed that her terrifying dreams would one day come true.

All the dreams had to do with her youngest brother. Her sixteen-year-old brother, Marti told me, had been tied to a bed since he was about two years old. Since the age of twelve, whenever he was untied, he would attack others or claw at himself. He spat at anyone who came close except his mother. Guttural, snarling sounds were his only methods of verbalization. He was unable to feed himself or control his bowel or bladder functions.

I was overwhelmed by Marti's disclosure. She continued her story.

Her brother had been the youngest of sixteen children, one of twins born to a mother almost fifty years old. The twin brother failed to thrive, and he died within weeks of birth. Some months thereafter, this surviving twin developed a seizure after suffering a high fever. He had convulsions regularly, which the family believed to be the result of witchcraft.

A medicine woman told the parents that the boy's umbilical cord had not been properly cut and disposed of. Through that improperly prepared stump, someone had transferred into him his twin brother's sickness. He could get well only if his dead brother's spirit were removed.

The medicine woman performed a ritual cleansing of Twin Boy, then burned things to help in the purification and the exorcism. She tied prayer feathers to his limbs. The mother too was told to cleanse herself. She was to shampoo her hair with special soap, drink a special tea, and not eat meat for some time.

Twin Boy did well for a while, but his seizures came harder. By two years of age, he required physical restraints because he banged his head, arms, and legs against hard objects. His family wondered if his twin brother was still within. The medicine woman said he might always be.

Twin Boy was never still. He would bang his head and eyes bloody. His mother remained devoted to him, sitting and playing with him for hours, restraining him only when he became self-mutilative and punched or bit himself.

His mother pleaded with the family not to mention Twin Boy's existence to authorities for fear that they would take him away; and after his infant immunizations, he never saw a doctor again. After all, the fever had first come after one such baby shot. In a way, she believed that his sickness was a curse that Twin Boy and she must live with. If the medicine woman's cures didn't work, there probably was no cure.

After the restraints became necessary all the time, the mother spoon-fed the boy. Later she would simply put the food close to his head where he ate it without using his hands. He could laugh, smile, and cry out, but he had never spoken a coherent word. Over the last several years the boy's frame had become deformed. He developed a severe hunchback. Still, the family kept his existence secret.

Marti now found it harder to accept the situation. Her mother was getting older and sickly. If she died, what would they do with Twin Boy? Marti felt she had to share the family secret with someone who would not laugh at her. The guilt, the shame, and the anger now were hurting her.

I asked her what I could do, and unhesitatingly she asked me to go see Twin Boy. I told her that I would come, but that she had to tell the other members of the family about my visit.

Marti not only made the announcement, but she told them that for the last two years she had been having bad dreams — so bad that she couldn't sleep and had no appetite. These dream thoughts had affected her at work, she told them, and she found herself crying at her desk. Marti explained that I told her she suffered from an illness that could be cured only by acknowledging the truth.

The family's relief was astounding. It seems that each member had been waiting for someone to offer an end to their shared suffering. By the time I rattled out there in the back of a truck, they were ready to consider alternatives.

I climbed out of the truck and walked with the family to an outside arbor under which Twin Boy lay. He was tied by all four extremities to a steel-cornered bed. Even from a distance I could see his hunchback. As I came closer, he snarled and spat at me. His fingers and eyes were mutilated; his teeth were decayed. I was speechless.

In the house, I explained to the family that maybe the time had come to think about what else could be done for Twin Boy. If they wanted, I would help find a place for him. The family already knew what needed to be done.

When Twin Boy first went into residential treatment, his mother stayed with him. The staff said that she related to him with extraordinary tenderness. He never snarled at her. One day she tearfully told Twin Boy that she was going, but that he would not be going with her. She knew that he understood he would never see her again.

The therapists and caretakers at this particular facility are highly trained and committed to their work. They helped this terribly disturbed child to become more self-sufficient. He became toilet-trained and learned to feed himself. He learned to bounce on a trampoline and to walk. Twin Boy even understood the token economy system in the home, whereby he got tokens he could redeem for candy when he performed well.

After the placement, someone entertained the idea of a lawsuit against the family for child abuse. I testified that when we take steps to confront serious human problems there are many ways to dance. Not only was the family committed to Twin Boy, but he had irreversible brain damage, and their care of him had saved the state at least three-quarters of a million dollars.

Twin Boy's family did not believe doctors could make him well, and as a matter of fact it may well have been a doctor who made him sick. His illness may have been a complication of DPT immunization, one of those one-in-a-million reactions to the shot.

The family chose to face their problem and care for this child themselves for as long as they could and in the best way they knew how. They had asked for help only when the mother had become old and enfeebled. There was no abuse here.

It's true that if Twin Boy had been placed early in his life in a superb institution like the one he was in now, he might have been helped to develop more quickly and fully. But, I argued, generally speaking, for one this profoundly impaired, being tied to a bed on the Apache reservation with the loving attention of his mother was better than being placed in most caretaking institutions in the United States.

The Tomato Lady

Della was a twenty-two-year-old Blackfeet woman from Montana, whose husband had died six months prior to her seeing me. A Mexican migrant worker, he was following the seasonal harvests when they met and married. They had lived in a town just off the reservation where Indians are still called "prairie niggers." He had been killed in a car wreck, driving drunk, two months before Della was to deliver their first baby.

Della brought Tesay, the baby girl, to Phoenix to get away from drunks of every description, including those in her family. She was significantly depressed when she came to see me. She raged against booze and her dead husband. After several months, she began to emerge from her deep depression.

I lost track of her for several years until one day she re-materialized in my office, terrified, chain-smoking cigarettes, and telling this story.

She was living with a man who was good to her and her daughter, but she had done a terrible thing. She had spent about three thousand dollars of what little money they had to have a psychic take away a curse.

Eight months before, at a county fair, she had received a "reading" for one dollar. The psychic had said that Della was in danger of repeating old mistakes that could destroy her. Della admitted that she was struggling with whether or not to get married. The psychic said she had already told Della too much. If Della wanted more details, she would have to see her at her office and she gave Della her card. Della could hardly wait until that evening to call for an appointment.

The following day, at the reading, the psychic told her that two people were conspiring to destroy her. They had paid a powerful witch to curse her. But if Della paid her five thousand dollars, then the psychic could prevent this disaster from happening. Della was not to tell anyone, the woman added. If she did, then Tesay, her daughter, might die.

"Bring part of the money to our next appointment, and also bring a tomato that you have rubbed all over your body," the psychic told her.

Della withdrew over a thousand dollars from the bank as an initial installment on the curse removal program. At her next visit to the psychic, the woman placed the tomato on a white handkerchief. She ordered Della to lay the large-denomination bills crosswise underneath it, then asked her to examine the tomato to see that there were no marks or blemishes on it.

After Della had completed the inspection, the psychic knotted the handkerchief and chanted over the bundle for God to help lift the curse from Della. She opened the bundle and had Della again confirm that there were no marks on the tomato. Then she split open the tomato. Inside was small, wooden head with real human hair. Blood dripped from its eyes and mouth.

As Della screamed in fear, the psychic asked if she wanted that to happen to her. "You must visit me regularly. I can make the curse disappear."

Not wishing to provoke such power further, Della began forking over payments on biweekly visits until she had given the psychic three thousand dollars, almost all that she had. When she finally told her boyfriend of the terrible dilemma, he was flabbergasted. He tried to sympathize with Della's fears, but his sympathy did not extend to his wallet. He adamantly refused to allow her to give the psychic another dime.

That was when Della came to me. She was terrified that the Tomato Lady had the power to seek retribution for her failure to complete her payments.

And what of the curse? Could that be reactivated against her? And now that she had told her boyfriend and me about the Tomato Lady, would the Tomato Lady make some disaster befall Tesay, as she had threatened? In desperation, Della asked me if I had a power greater than that of the psychic.

"Yes," I told her. "I have a power. You have power too."

Before she could puzzle that through, I shouted at her: "Give me your car keys! Right now. Give them here!"

Della was surprised by my sudden outburst. "Give you my keys?" she asked. "Why should I give you my keys?"

"I want your car!" I screamed. "Give me your keys!"

"But . . ."

"Don't question me!" I scowled at her. "Do as I tell you."

Although she seemed genuinely frightened by my strange behavior, Della stood her ground. "Why should I give you my keys?"

After a long silence, I asked, "Why did you give your keys to the Tomato Lady?"

In Della's confusion, I continued: "Not your *car* keys. But you gave her the keys to your personal power. The greatest power we have is the power to make choices. If you give someone the keys to your car, then you can't complain where they drive it. If you give someone the keys of responsibility for your happiness, then you can't complain if they don't make you happy."

How do we get the power to choose? We take it. It's almost as easy to exercise that power as it is to give it away. Doctors are vehicles for self-empowerment.

Indians try to look into the heart of a doctor to decide whether or not to come to him or her. The doctor must convince them that he or she has the power to heal. To accomplish this, the doctor must learn the many ways one can change the ordinary into the mystical, not just the opposite.

The melody you sing, like the steps you dance, is less important than the power of the connection your song establishes. The connection helps the patient heal. Della invested me with more power to heal than the Tomato Lady had power to harm. I was able to help her regain her own power. It doesn't matter how you do it, only that you do it.

Chapter 10

 # A KIDNAPPING
AND PAGE: CHILDREN

A Kidnapping

"Newborn Infant Kidnapped!"

The newspaper reported that a baby had been abducted from the Tuba City Indian Hospital in northern Arizona. A two-day-old male infant had disappeared, and someone had been seen walking out of the hospital with him. When they found the perpetrator two days later, she quickly admitted her guilt. The public defender sent her to see me, in hopes of establishing an insanity defense.

Dorothy, the young woman who had taken the baby, had been born to a mother who had not wanted her. She still did not know who her father was. As an infant, Dorothy had been given to her grandmother, who raised her in a small traditional village. She saw her mother rarely, and when she did come, her mother always referred to Dorothy as a sister. In the Navajo way, this rejection was serious and it always reminded Dorothy that she was unwanted.

But her grandmother loved her. She taught Dorothy to cook, weave, and participate in ceremonies, and the two of them became very close. When she was fourteen, Dorothy decided to get married, which is not so unusual in traditional

Navajoland after one boy keeps coming around regularly. From the earliest days of the marriage, Dorothy wanted a baby, but she could not get pregnant.

Six years after her marriage and now living in Phoenix, Dorothy learned during an outpatient visit to the hospital that she was pregnant for the first time. Her ecstasy was beyond words. She bought maternity clothes and started wearing them just to show everyone the wonderfulness of her condition. Her husband was as delighted as she. At last she would have her baby, and she would give it all that she wished had been given to her.

Five months into the pregnancy, in midwinter, her grandmother became ill and asked Dorothy for help. There was no way that Dorothy could deny the one person who had always been kind to her. She returned to the reservation to chop wood, help haul hay, and fetch groceries for her grandmother.

On the second night there, Dorothy awoke with cramping in her abdomen. She rushed to the bathroom and was horrified to discover that she had miscarried. In her hand, she held the precious but now deceased male fetus.

Dorothy crept out into the night and buried the fetus under a tree in the old way. The next morning she continued her errands. She met some relatives, but she told no one what had happened.

As she drove back to Phoenix a couple of days later, Dorothy's head was filled with one thought: she couldn't go home without a baby. What would she say to her husband? Did the miscarriage mean she was unable ever to be a mother? Why was she being deprived of this one thing that she so desperately wanted and deserved?

Dorothy had to come home with a baby. She could not think about anything else. In Flagstaff she bought some clothing for a baby and a striped blouse for herself. She made a plan that, in her obsessed state of mind, made perfect sense.

Dorothy drove on to the hospital in Tuba City. There she learned the names of some new mothers and chose one who had just given birth to a son. Wearing a candy-striped blouse and claiming to be a photographer's assistant, Dorothy asked the woman if she wanted some pictures taken of the baby. When the mother agreed, Dorothy picked the baby up from the mother's side and left the room. She kept walking to her pickup truck and drove off. That simply, Dorothy had her baby. She stopped to buy bottled formula, then continued to Phoenix.

At home, her husband and friends marveled at how big the baby was for such a short gestation, but a spirit of celebration prevailed. They bought clothes, gave the baby a name, and proudly showed him off. For two days, everyone could see that Dorothy was at last a mother. Later she learned that the name she and her husband gave the child was quite close to what the biological parents named him.

After her arrest and evaluation, Dorothy was released on her own recognizance. Her family held a ceremony for her. Everyone in her extended family was willing to share some responsibility toward the resolution of the event. In the Navajo way, when something bad happens to someone in a family or clan, it casts a pall over all the members, which the relatives then marshal forces to get rid of. This tradition is a classic example of community psychiatry, or family therapy, or systems therapy, whatever you want to call it. All promote the idea of bringing many forces together to best mobilize the powers that promote health.

Dorothy knew that she was not alone when her natural mother came to her during the ceremony and, for the first time, called her "daughter." At the baby's christening, his biological family prayed for forgiveness for the kidnapper, and then invited her to be godparent to the child. In this way, they offered forgiveness. Later, the child's family asked Dorothy and her people to join them on Mother's Day. They went, bringing a slaughtered sheep to share.

By the time Dorothy's case came to trial, both parties were satisfied with the healing and forgiveness the families had made possible. My testimony explained that both parties understood that unconscious forces controlled Dorothy's mind at the time of the kidnapping, and that at that moment she was powerless to do otherwise. She did not have a criminal mind and there was little likelihood that such an act would happen again. The charge was reduced to burglary. Dorothy was given a probationary term.

The families had made peace, and Dorothy had begun to find, through her family's love, a power that could balance the strength of her desire for a child. We could learn something from their experience.

Page

Kee and Desbah's six-month-old son had developed meningitis. On their way to the hospital in Page, they stopped to participate in an all-night ceremony—maybe a medicine man could cure him. But after the ceremony the baby was still in respiratory distress, so they continued their journey to Page. They planned to call a pediatrician they had once visited there.

In the emergency room, their doctor's associate was on duty and he examined the baby. Seeming annoyed by their presence, he scowled at the couple and pointedly asked them why they had not come to the hospital sooner. Kee and Desbah felt uneasy at the doctor's unfriendly reception, but they answered truthfully that they had stopped on the way to see a medicine man.

The doctor went into a rage. The two Navajos could not have angered him more if they had announced their memberships in a lobby for socialized medicine or in a cult whose members drank the blood of humans. "It will be your fault if your child dies!" he exploded. "You should have come sooner!"

Kee and Desbah literally staggered from this accusation as if the doctor had physically struck them. Navajo parents do not kill their sick children. The very thought was incomprehensible to them.

They left the child at the hospital, but the following morning they came to request the doctor to transfer the case to another physician; they didn't think this angry man could help their child. The doctor refused to see them.

Kee and Desbah felt they had only one choice—they must take their baby out of this hospital.

A nurse called the doctor and told him that the parents intended to remove the patient from hospital care. She hung up the phone and looked at them. "The doctor told me to tell you that your baby will die without the medicines of the hospital," the nurse told Kee and Desbah. "He says that you must leave the baby here."

"We have no choice," Kee told the nurse.

Desbah added firmly, "The doctor does not feel good about us. How can he feel good about our baby? We will take our child to the Indian hospital in Tuba City."

On the way to the Indian hospital, Kee and Desbah stopped again at the house of the medicine man for a blessing. He looked at the child and told them to take him straight to the hospital. By the time they arrived, their baby was dead.

Criminal charges of involuntary manslaughter were filed against Kee and Desbah. The doctor at Page testified that, in his opinion, the parents were responsible for the death of their child.

During his deposition, the doctor was asked if, when he first saw the parents in the emergency room, he had said hello or introduced himself. He could not remember. He was then asked if he had told them that it would be their fault if the baby died. He did remember that. He also conceded that he was angry and it had probably showed.

With the help of an interpreter, the parents told the court that they believed healing required the proper spirit. There had to be mutual trust among the healer, patient, and family. The doctor had not inspired their trust; he had humiliated them and implied that they would harm their child. They believed their baby would not survive in his hands. When he had refused to speak with them, they felt they had no other choice.

In my deposition, I explained that from the Navajo perspective it is unthinkable for any healer to believe that he or she alone does the healing. All parties—the spiritual source, the family, the clan, the patient and the medicine man—were participants in the healing process. To overemphasize one's singular importance and to denigrate that of others did not inspire confidence. This doctor blamed the family for their baby's condition; how could they believe in his healing power?

The case was eventually dropped. Hoping to avert a similar tragedy in the future, I wrote to the doctor and the hospital administration, offering to talk, free of charge, about traditional healing practices. In part, my letter stated:

> From the Navajo perspective, healing is a shared responsibility between patient and doctor. There must be a sense of commitment, belief, and harmony among all parties. Your experience with one another deemphasized such a harmonious exchange. It was a relationship of inequality in which the parents believed themselves humiliated. Hurt and angry, they returned to their own people and healers.
>
> Page lies in the midst of Navajo country and serves a large Indian population. The degree to which we can sensitize ourselves to the needs and beliefs of our constituents, even if we do not share those beliefs, will determine how we might better provide for their health needs.

I never received a response.

Chapter 11

POPEYE AND SOLOHO

The White Mountains of Arizona contain some of the most beautiful natural scenery in the world. Trout-filled streams cross meadows; forests of ponderosa pine lead to snow-capped peaks. The land sustains elk, bear, and mountain lion. The White Mountain Apaches own and operate a popular ski resort and a profitable lumber mill.

The name "Apache" conjures up silver-screen images of warriors in breechcloths, of cavalry forts and wily Geronimo. This is a people with whom the United States government only made peace in the 1900s. They are the last defeated Indian nation in this country, and they fought almost to the last man to keep their freedom. The concept of a reservation was entirely foreign to the wandering Apaches, who traveled over the hills and canyons of southeastern Arizona in hunting and warring bands of twenty or thirty people. Today's Apaches are quite disconnected from that colorful past. Nothing has replaced those old ways to give the Apache the same sense of pride and power.

I once asked a group of three- and four-year-old Indian Head Start students to draw a picture of their community. The children drew the usual houses, streets, stores, and schools. Interspersed among the buildings were stick figures. When I asked what the stick figures were doing, the children said, "Those are people lying around."

"What are they doing?" I asked.

The children answered, "They're drunk."

Even by the age of three, children accept this prevalence of alcoholism as ordinary. Alcohol, not the cavalry, may sow the final seeds of extinction among the Apache.

Whiteriver, in the heart of the White Mountains, is Popeye's home. Born to a mother who died of liver failure when he was a year old, Popeye was adopted by a white family and left the reservation.

He had a happy childhood and loved his family. Popeye got his nickname because he clapped his hands and gurgled when he heard the cartoon's theme song on television. He had a natural instinct for music. From early on, he banged rhythmically on any available surface or hummed with the windshield wipers. He learned to play the guitar, and he wrote songs.

In adolescence, Popeye joined the high-school Indian Club as he began to sort out his own identity issues. Although his parents openly dealt with his being Indian, they were unable to help him understand how it fit into who he was.

Popeye wanted to know about his biological mother. The adoption agency that had placed him gave him his mother's name, and he began to seek out what he could learn about her. On the reservation he met relatives who welcomed him back. As they offered him a beer, they told him about his mother's alcoholic death. Popeye spent some time with his relatives, but the drinking on the reservation was so overwhelming that he had to leave.

In his early twenties Popeye married his high-school sweetheart, a non-Indian. They had two sons, and he named each after an Apache chieftain. Popeye was proud of being Apache, and he wanted his sons to be proud too. He played guitar professionally while attending a local community college. The pace destroyed his marriage, he said later; he was just never around.

When I met Popeye, he was thirty years old and quadraplegic. This is how it happened.

At a party at a condominium, Popeye had gotten drunk and climbed onto a balcony that overlooked a central swimming pool. When he had everyone's attention, he announced that he was going to dive into the water. He did—and they had to drag him out. By the time the medics came, Popeye was barely breathing—another alcohol-related trauma, one of the so many Indian hospitals are besieged with.

A month later, when I first saw Popeye, he was depressed and withdrawn. He communicated only by screaming, primarily at the nurses. I said that I had come because the staff was concerned about how foul-mouthed and angry he was. He told me he didn't need a fucking shrink, and the litany began—"Bastard . . . fucker . . . white man . . . let me die! . . . The nurses stink . . . the government sucks . . ." and so on.

I went to my office to get a tape recorder and brought it back to his room. Popeye started his rap as soon as I hit the door. I switched the recorder on and left again. Fifteen minutes later I returned and replayed the tape for him. When the recording of his obscenities was over, Popeye screamed, "I hope you die. Because if you don't, I'll kill you!"

I yelled back. "Bullshit! It's just easier to get angry than to be afraid." I'd been there. Then I left.

Popeye stayed angry, but we talked. When he noticed movement in his shoulder, he started to mellow. A little later there was action in his arms and even his fingers and wrist. Now he wondered if he could beat it, how soon he could walk.

Popeye's attitude changed completely. No longer bitter and angry, he started talking about getting his fingers into better shape; he was going to make it in the music business. Now Popeye was laughing all the time, teasing the nurses, and talking about a marathon run.

I got suspicious. Was he denying reality and setting himself up for real disappointment?

I wanted to help him become more realistic about his crippled condition, so I asked him if he ever got mad or sad anymore.

"Yeah. I get mad whenever somebody reminds me that I'll spend the rest of my life in this goddamn wheelchair!"

A speechless moment. To me, Popeye's positive talk was not realistic. But so what? It was his life. My perception of reality is not necessarily the way it is. It's only the way I see it; it's just real for me. I didn't ask him to look at it my way again, not even when he told me he was going to be a marathoner.

For a long time I believed if you felt good because you were denying or minimizing realities, such feelings were based on illusions. Sooner or later the truth would come out, and you would be shattered along with your illusions. But there is intrinsic value to positive feelings, and I've learned that it's more effective to influence others using their perceptions of reality. I no longer tell patients how I see their reality unless they ask—and then I do so with considerable caution.

Psychologists using sophisticated tests have recently rediscovered this obvious fact: people who respond to a life-threatening illness with denial have a much better chance of surviving it. In all healing, the patient has a powerful impact on making it happen. Feeling or doing something positive can influence the outcome.

States of consciousness and awareness have a strong impact on the healing process. Current concepts of disease don't explain how, but these states can produce a change in one's level of physical functioning. Laughter can produce curative substances in the body; relaxation can lower blood pressure, increase blood flow, and raise skin temperature. You can change you brain rhythms; you can alter your perceptions of pain.

Science doesn't quite explain how this happens, but as a culture we share an urge for explanations. Indian healers understand that the questions are more important than the answers.

Herbert had introduced me to Bill Dalton, a Hopi healer, who lived in Whiteriver. It was from Bill that Herbert got his medicines. Bill had a controversial history and he seemed to have his share of detractors, but as he got older people sought him out. He liked to introduce himself by his Indian name, Soloho, the Whistling Arrow.

Bill's single-room cabin on the reservation was just large enough for a bed, a table, a wood-burning stove, and a foot locker filled with herbs. He was then in his seventies—vigorous, crinkled, a good-looking, good-humored old man who wore a headband over pageboy bangs.

When I met him he was skinning a mountain lion that had been deposited at his doorstep by the tribal trapper. After the greeting, I watched him, and he asked if I wanted a piece. It wasn't kosher, I told him, and he laughed and said

I couldn't use it anyway because it was more pussy than I could handle.

Years later, Bill told me about an experience in Hawaii where he treated a well-known singer who, for some reason, had been unable to perform. After Bill "worked on" him, he was able to go on stage that night. The story was publicized in the local paper, and some kahunas, native Hawaiian healers, invited him to attend a ceremony.

Not knowing what to expect, Bill went to the location. The kahunas blindfolded him and eventually led him up a mountainside into a cave where the blindfold was removed. Bill saw that he had crawled through a narrow passage leading into a chamber. In the middle of the cavern was a sunken pool into which steps had been carved. The kahunas chanted and moved their arms, just like Hopis do in certain ceremonies. The head kahuna took Bill to the pool's edge, and asked him to look at the water and tell what he saw.

Bill said he saw ripples that appeared almost as waves on the water's surface. The kahuna asked him to explain their presence.

Bill knew that he saw waves, that the waves were there, but he knew the mountain wasn't moving and that he was higher than sea level. He didn't know *why* there were waves, but he knew the kahuna had asked him an important question. So he answered: "I know there are waves, and I know they are important."

The head kahuna nodded and got undressed, motioning Bill to do so as well. Then they both walked down the stairs into the pool. Soloho's initiation was complete.

The riddle still escaped me, so I asked Bill what the answer was. He laughed and said, "You white people are all the same.

What's the answer? The kahunas didn't know the answer either. Some questions don't have answers. It's enough to know that the question is important."

What we see is not all there is; it's only as much as we can answer now. We will probably never know the whole story.

The kahunas only know that when the pool surface stops rippling, civilization will come to an end. *How* makes no real difference. It's important to recognize the value of questions and to accept the mystery. The willingness not to know it all allows us to be in touch with the more intuitive, creative, unbridled parts of ourselves.

Psychoanalytic theories are so preoccupied with biographical questions of why, how, when, where, that they lose sight of the fact that the answers don't change anything—and sometimes they even interfere.

Years later, I saw Popeye's picture in the newspaper. The caption explained that he was one of the participants to finish in a wheelchair marathon.

We are here for such a brief period of time. We come and go like flickers of a flame. Sometimes we get so serious about what it all means. The important thing is to play the hand you've been dealt.

The Indians take the perspective that death will take care of itself. The past and the future are simply reflections of an everlasting *now*. In this ongoing present reality, we are connected to those who came before and to those who will come after.

We are here to help each other discover our individual uniqueness. This selfhood, once understood, will of itself sustain us and will, in turn, connect us to the larger reality of humans and spiritual experience. In that way, we may all become dancing healers.

Chapter 12

 HEALING

When I came to Indian country as a young doctor, I thought I was bringing truth, healing, and knowledge to a backward people. In those first years, I was sometimes met with anger and hostility, other times with indifference. Even the patients who "needed" me the most seemed to shrug their shoulders at my explanations of what could and could not be done to heal them.

I am a better healer now. I have learned that the patient doesn't need a scientist who simply carries out instructions from the laboratory manual. Patients don't want to be cases— they want to be healed. They want to participate in their own wellness or their own death. Patients are the principal agents in their lives, and as much as they want to be well, they want peace and understanding. To find such a healing peace they need to feel that a connection exists between themselves and the healer and between themselves and something larger than self or science.

What patients believe about the doctor's ability to heal may make the difference in their recovery. It certainly makes a difference in their peace of mind.

As I've continued my quest to become a healer, I've learned many steps from many dancers. It is through these steps that I have become a better doctor, a better psychiatrist. As I've learned to share the steps of others I've discovered my own music. I've learned more about being human and about faith.

We are always patients, and sometimes we are healers. We move from being one to being the other. Sometimes I do the work, and sometimes someone else does the work.

Here are some of my own stories. I hope my mentors will smile at my dance. They have taught me the steps.

"Primitive" Indian cultures have used many powerful natural substances as sacraments. Modern culture tends to abuse these same substances: alcohol, tobacco, hallucinogens, herbs.

The special tobacco the Navajo or the Plains tribes smoke in ceremonies is a mixture of herbs and native tobacco that has meaning for its role in ritual. The smoke gives color and smell to one's words. What is said can be sent on the wings of an eagle to touch God's ear. And the smoke can cleanse the body of the clinging dust of ordinary reality. The power of the smoke comes from mixing your breath with that of others, a reminder that we are all on this path together—people, plants, animals, and air.

The smoke is not "funny" tobacco, and the ritual has nothing to do with smoking cigarettes compulsively. Addiction is the opposite of sacrament. Nothing could be less sacred than consuming a substance habitually until it becomes ordinary and no longer has its special power.

Herbs too have a place in the sacrament of healing, as do

singing songs, burning cedar, waving feathers, holding teddy bears, or any other sign of hope.

Joe, a middle-aged Chippewa traditionalist, built a sweat lodge on his wife's reservation (in spite of the community's disapproval) and used it regularly as a way of dealing with a chronic abdominal pain. He worked as a long-distance truck driver until he decided that if he were to cramp while driving, the danger to himself and others would be too great. He quit driving, but he couldn't stand working inside, and he needed to be his own boss. "Just tell me where you want it; I'll get it there" was as much supervision as he tolerated.

Unable to drive his truck, Joe didn't know what else to do. More accurately, he *believed* there was nothing else he could do. He was afraid to explore other paths, in part because he had dropped out of school and he feared that technical training would require more effort than he believed he could expend.

He was referred to me by the internists who told him they had done all they could for his abdominal cramps. He had heard something about me and he knew I wouldn't judge his sweat lodge practices as peculiar.

He told me his story—about a large abusive family, delinquency, running away, and other run-ins. He had returned to the traditional spiritual path during an incarceration. He had been doing well, was working, and was committed to his family until he got sick.

After listening to his story, I did not interpret Joe's concerns about competence, fear, intelligence, or masculinity. Instead, I had him imagine a voyage inside his abdomen to the afflicted spot. In his imagination, he could breathe in a healing, flexible fiberoptic light, carried in an illuminated air bubble, and allow it to course through his body from his lungs through his heart and into his abdomen, right to the place of pain.

And he saw the pain as an ugly, dark, baseball-sized mass that had an irregular margin with a piece reaching out like a finger. He visualized the finger as a dark tunnel with him inside. He could see a light at its end. I told Joe he would be guided through the tunnel by a source of power that would come to him as an animal.

He saw a giant green moth, of a species that had flown near his childhood home. This creature led him to the light.

Afterwards, I told him that a moth is an interesting animal. It starts out life as an animal that crawls, then it changes and gets wings and becomes an animal that flies. Nothing stays the same. You start rolling and then discover you can fly. He also understood that the green moth was his power animal, and he could use it and depend on it to give him strength, because it was his; it was himself. He could fly.

I also gave Joe some herbs for his stomach recommended by an herbalist, an Anglo woman married to a Navajo, who gathers herbs from untouched places in the desert and sells them all over the world.

Finally, I offered to give him some leads about career counseling and vocational testing, which he accepted a short time later. He did get another job, and he found there was another way to move. And finally his pains disappeared.

People always provide keys like the moth; all of us have the keys to our own enlightenment. The therapist uses whatever symbols mean something to that patient. Patients already have the answers to their questions. As the therapist listens to the problem, the patient will also tell the solution.

When you choose to take the journey of enlightenment, you always find guides. And nothing is so big that you do not already have the resources to meet it.

What we see as science, the Indians see as magic. What we see as magic, they see as science. I don't find this a hopeless contradiction. If we can appreciate each other's views, we can see the whole picture more clearly. To heal ourselves or to help heal others we need to reconnect magic and science, our right and left brains.

Mainstream America is a left-brain culture—we believe in rational scientific thought, causality, explanation. The right brain is the home of magic, of intuition, emotion, creativity, faith, the irrational. Great discoveries in science or art are made through the nonrational, nonlinear insights of the right brain. It is the left brain that knows how to speak, but the right brain that remembers the lyrics to songs. You need both sides to dance. You need both sides to remain healthy.

More and more, psychiatry emphasizes the left brain and the biochemical explanations for all behavior, without equal effort to understand the magic and mystering of healing. And it's the healing that matters, not the techniques or the explanations.

The Indian healers' methods are based in faith, but when their methods don't work, they never hesitate to send a suffering person to a hospital or a white doctor. They use whatever works.

Healing is what works.

Flora was a Mexican-Yaqui woman who had been raised in a series of foster homes. She was repeatedly sexually abused and raped in two of her foster homes. Her mother was said to be a witch, and Flora believed her mother could cast spells. She was afraid to go home, even for a short time.

By the time I met Flora, she had some serious psychiatric problems and relied on pills to remain on an even keel. She had also managed to earn a master's degree and was working as a health professional. Flora was articulate; she presented her history undefensively and was capable of listening, so she was an excellent psychotherapy candidate.

Her most significant breakthrough occurred during a Yaqui Easter ceremony. It was the mystical Indian part of her that seemed to hold some power over Flora. She knew the symbology of the Yaquis' Easter rituals and at some level she believed in their power.

Over several weeks during the holy season, members of the Yaqui tribe enact an elaborate ritual that combines elements of their original Indian faith and the Catholic beliefs they learned from missionaries. On the day before Easter, there is a symbolic burning of a cloth-draped wooden statue of Judas. The statue is paraded into the courtyard in front of the community's Catholic church. The figure is surrounded by musicians and revelers wearing human and animals masks and jingling leg rattles. They are the chapayekas, Judas's entourage, and they are rejoicing over his betrayal of Christ.

But soon Judas will be torched, and the forces of goodness will obliterate the evil and the age of salvation will be born. The ritual not only replicates the Christian story; it also gives participants an opportunity to give up some of their old sins, conflicts, fears, or pains in a symbolic way. People tie offerings of hope and relief to the Judas figure.

Flora did not want to participate in the ceremony, because she did not want to confront her mother. So I told her I would take the offering for her. Flora brought me a scarf of hers and as we talked about her life, she used the scarf to wipe her tears.

I went to the Saturday ceremony at the Yaqui village of Guadalupe. At the appropriate time, I tied Flora's tear-stained scarf carrying her painful history and my hope for her relief to the Judas figure. No one stopped or questioned me; no one stops seekers from realizing their hope. As the Judas burned, I felt, in addition to the horror, a sense of hope, even awe, at the power of this setting.

Flora's healing came equally from the burning of her tear-stained past and from my tying it to the Judas. In addition to the negative force of her mother's power, she had an even stronger conviction that she could find relief. Her belief was bolstered by the knowledge that I had taken it all seriously enough to perform the ritual. Flora did much better; she soon left the state, and left much of her painful past behind.

Walking the path together promotes the healing process.

One of my patients was a twenty-year-old Anglo woman, the daughter of a dear friend. Less than six months after her marriage, a large inoperable tumor was discovered in her neck. A cancer of the lymph glands, it extended into her chest. It was responsive to chemo- and radiotherapy, but the chemicals made Tracy sick; even the smells in the oncologist's waiting room made her throw up.

Tracy's husband and family tried to get her to take the treatments, but she felt too weak. She spent her days watching television soap operas, interrupted only for appointments with the radiation therapist. Finally, her mother-in-law prevailed on her at least to talk to someone outside the family, hoping someone would convince Tracy to go for chemotherapy.

But Tracy's agenda was different. She didn't want the chemotherapy now. She was skeletal, jaundiced, weak, and she wanted to know what I believed. Did I believe, as she did, that this would pass and then she would be okay?

I talk about these things now—not just what the patient believes, but also what I believe, how I understand the mysterious.

Tracy talked about childhood friends and the ocean and her wedding picture and her dog. During these days, Tracy imagined this peaceful scene: she saw herself as a little girl in a meadow of flowers and clover, with protective trees. She could visualize a rickety bridge leading over a creek. The other side was not clear, but she could cross the bridge, and if she felt frightened she could hold onto supports around her. The rail was her husband's hand, and her grandmother's, and her dog was beside her on the way.

I said that each life is a series of bridges. We cross new ones as we move from one life phase to another. Sometimes the bridges reach over chasms of pain, of fear, or of sadness. And the only way to make it across is to be supported by something that reminds you that you are not alone.

In her peaceful meadow, Tracy once rode on the back of a giant eagle and soared above the bridge to look at the dark side. It was less forbidding than she had feared. When the great bird landed she saw herself dismounting into the hands of loved ones.

I shared my beliefs and values with Tracy. I talked about my own pain and my own connections. I sang to her in Hebrew and English a song of the Hasidic master, Reb Nachman of Bratislav. He taught that the unknown is an adventure, and the way to make it through was not to fear.

> The whole world is just a narrow bridge.
> Just a narrow bridge, and
> Above all, above all,
> Is not to fear,
> Not to fear, at all.

Eight weeks after I first saw Tracy she died. She had kept the tape of my song and stories at her bedside. She played it twice a day to help her rest. I feel as good about giving her this as I would as if I had been able to persuade her to go for chemotherapy.

My old Jewish connections keep coming back to me. Every time I think I've got my identity clear, something happens to remind me of those connections. I had been raised in a conservative, if not absolutely observant, Jewish home. As a young man I rejected this part of my past because it didn't have all the answers. In the radicalism of the 1960s, many of us dismissed any and all traditions in an attempt to free ourselves from hypocrisy—we threw the baby out with the bath.

In Santa Fe, I tried to raise my children with the consciousness of universalists, as members of the tribe of humankind. They would learn to believe in the unity of humankind, not to follow restrictive practices of one tribe.

Then one day the children decided they wanted to go to church with their friends in this very Catholic town. I suddenly rediscovered the force of my attachment to the old connection. This happened at the same time that I was learning another dance from the Pueblos and the power of their connections. The reality hit me: my children didn't know what they were. They didn't really know what it meant to be a Jew. I discovered that it mattered to me what they were, what I was. It was a connection of truth and one of credibility. This is my tribe. So we began going to the synagogue again. In the absence of our circuit-riding rabbi, I even filled in for him a few times.

All tribes, all religions, are sustained by similar myths — births, rebirths, faith in miracles. These stories, these connections to our way, are the predicates on which all morality is based. They are what sustains us as good people in the hard times. I came to realize that you have to know who you are before you can be a universalist; it's what makes us each unique that lets us appreciate the universalities among us. If you can realize that your heritage is part of what makes you special, then you can realize that others are special too.

In time, however, I found organized Jewish worship a difficult place to feel the spirit. The synagogue was the least spiritual place I knew. On the holiest days, great throngs and multiple distractions made it hard to be serious about prayer. It was in the tipi or the sweat lodge that I was best able to see the face of Abraham, to huddle with Jacob in the desert, to feel the presence of a spirit in the coals of a fire.

Lately a small group of friends and I have spent these holy days creating our own liturgy. We prepare ourselves for the penance of the Days of Awe in our own sweat lodge. It is built with the traditional frame of twelve willow branches; I see them as the tribes of Israel.

In the circle, we pass sacred objects and each participant talks. We recall our desert ancestry and our connections to the Earth. We sing the old melodies, we burn cedar, we recreate in the small group a circle of faith, a place of prayer. Prayer is an expression of the heart that goes directly to the tongue without first being short-circuited by the brain.

Every day, in many ways, in unexpected places, you can hear a new tune and learn another step in your dance.

Chapter 13

THE SUN DANCE

I first heard about Brave Buffalo from Basil, my Phoenix Indian High School friend who, after graduation, became involved in the American Indian Movement. After participating in marches and military confrontations for a time, he found himself on the Indian spiritual path—the "Red Road." He became involved with a traditional Indian spiritual community in Portland, Oregon, called Anpo, the Lakota Sioux word for "dawn."

Anpo is a realization of the vision of Brave Buffalo, a Brule Sioux. The community conducts Indian-sensitive teaching programs for the Portland public schools; it sponsors museum exhibitions, dances, and craft fairs. Brave Buffalo has lectured about traditional Indian beliefs all over America and Europe. He has a fifth-grade education, but he has much to say.

Once a year, in July (the Moon of Making Fat), Brave Buffalo sponsors a Sun Dance. He had a dream telling him to recreate the sacred hoop of the Sun Dance, the most sacred ceremony of the Plains tribes, which include the Sioux.

If you have a vision and believe in its validity, you have to do what it commands. You have to share it with others;

otherwise it's like a gift that remains forever unopened.

For the last four years, Anpo has sponsored a Sun Dance on grounds in the Mt. Hood National Forest. The Forest Service closes the area to other users during the four days of the ceremony.

The participants in the Sun Dance believe that if Indian people come together again in this sacred circle, civilization will endure. If they fulfill this commitment made by their ancestors to Wakan Tanka, the Great Spirit, then the earth will survive.

The dancers dance not for themselves alone, but for their families, their tribes, and for all of humankind. As a gesture of surrender to the Creator, warriors pierce their flesh with sticks. They believe their flesh is the only thing they can offer to the Creator that is truly their own.

Black Elk, the Sioux visionary and Keeper of the Sacred Pipe, spoke of the Sun Dance in this way:

> We hold it during the Moon of Making Fat, because this is the time when the sun is at its highest and the growing power of the world is strongest. We select the sacred tree. The people come to it singing, with flowers all over them. A brave warrior strikes the living tree, counting coup on it [from the practice in warfare of hitting a fallen enemy with a stick, which then counted him as a casualty], because the spirit of the sun loves everything that bears fruit. Then maidens chop it down. We carry it home, stopping four times, once for each season and direction, to give thanks for this gift of life. Then the sacred tree is set down at a place in the center. We plant it in the earth; we make a vow to the Great Spirit, Wakan Tanka.
>
> This tree is the center of the living universe. It holds the power of the world. It is the centerpiece of the four

directions. The East brings peace and light; the South, warmth; the West brings rain; and the North, strength and endurance.

The sky is the great circle that surrounds us. The earth is the circle that supports us. The sun comes and goes in a great circle just like our lives.

Everything in life is a great circle; the tipis are round like the nests of birds—they hold the children who are the guardians of our immortality. And we are, in turn, embraced by the Earth Mother who in her roundness provides us with the fruitfulness of life.

On the morning before the Sun Dance, nursing mothers bring their little ones to be blessed at the base of the tree of life, here at the center of the universe. Grow up and be brave; make your people proud.

Holy men will pierce their ears. The dancers paint their bodies; they lay beneath the tree and the holy men cut places in their backs or chest so they can fulfill their oaths. Each man thus fastened to the tree gets up and dances until his flesh tears loose.

This is the dancers' pledge: I give you this piece of my spirit, give me the peace of your presence. I touch your presence on this Mother Earth; treat me with kindness and give my people life.

By the beginning of the twentieth century, the Sun Dance had been outlawed as a barbaric ritual. The offering of living flesh as a sacrifice was deemed a degenerate and primitive practice. The Sioux later petitioned the courts, saying that fulfilling this sacred obligation was necessary to ensure their lives, indeed the lives of everyone on earth. Eventually, the government relented and permitted the Sun Dance—but without piercing. With the passage of the Native American Religious Freedoms Act in 1978 public piercing was again allowed.

When I attended the Sun Dance, I thought I'd be one of the few non-Indians. It turns out there were Germans, French, Japanese, Rastafarians, Christians, Jews, Mormons, and Buddhists. Mostly, there were Indian people from tribes all over the hemisphere—hundreds of people, all together for this seeking of the spirit.

The sacred grounds look like an Edward Curtis photograph of nineteenth-century Indian life. A semicircle of tipis surrounds the Sacred Hoop. At the center, inside a branch-covered arbor, stands the Sun Dance pole; it's about fifty feet high and draped with scarves of red, white, yellow, and black, the colors of the four directions.

Wrapped around the trunk are ropes, one for each dancer who has tied his own spiritual lifeline to the tree. Once he ties the rope, it has to be used, otherwise his spirit can't be released. If a dancer becomes sick or for some other reason can't be pierced, someone else must complete the ritual for him. At the very top of the tree an eagle feather and two leather figurines, one, a man, the other a buffalo, both danced in the breeze.

Surrounding the pole, at a radius of maybe fifty feet, is a covered arbor under which all the supporters stand, except at the open east end of the circle. Dawn's first ray must strike the sacred tree unobstructed.

At the western edge of the arbor is a covered ramada where the dancers rest between dance rounds. Behind it is an enclosed compound with three tipis and sweat lodges. The dancers stay in the compound without eating or drinking for four days.

They enter the sweat lodges twice daily. Even after four days, they still sweat. I don't know how they do it with no fluid intake. In medical school, I was taught that the body could not survive without water after three days because the kidneys start to shut down.

After days of prayer and preparation, the Sun Dance begins at dawn. Everyone is called to the arbor by a raucous symphony of eagle-bone whistles. Each dancer wears a whistle around his neck and blows it while moving. I hear the cry in my sleeping bag and feel like a target in Alfred Hitchcock's movie *The Birds*.

The first to enter the circle is a Horned Buffalo Dancer; he carries a "smudge pot," a number-10 can filled with burning sage; he brushes the smoke into the arbor with an eagle feather to sanctify the place and its occupants. All present are now in the center of all things. This cleansing ritual separates us from every influence outside the circle: from the worries, pain, antagonisms, and ordinary fears of daily life, from all except the feeling of the spirit within the hoop.

Pregnant women are welcomed under the arbor because this place is a good influence on unborn children, but menstruating women are not allowed into the circle. They are not excluded in shame, but in recognition of their special power and influence at this time.

At the south side of the circle is the great drum. Its rhythms behind the chanted melodies captivate us with their vibrations. My feet move; my body sways. The songs says, "Wakan Tanka—Great Spirit—here we are at the center; we have only you in our minds."

Following the Buffalo Dancer comes a woman cradling the sacred pipe. She represents the White Buffalo Calf Woman who originally brought the sacred pipe to the people and instructed them in its use.

Into the red pipestone bowl is carved a figure of the sacred buffalo, the bringer of all goodness, which fed, clothed, housed, and sustained the people. Beneath the bowl is an eagle feather for the sacred brother whose wings touch the ear of the Creator, Wakan Tanka, the bringer of light. Tied to the pipe's shaft are sage and sweet grass, a reminder that if the people bind themselves to the Spirit in this sacred way, then they will multiply and the earth endure.

The Lakota smoke the pipe whenever they conduct sacred business. The pipe ceremony prepares any setting for truth. Like the smoke smudging, it separates the ordinary from the extraordinary, the profane from the sacred. When you share the smoke, the breath of your life spirit, with others in the spirit of truth, something good will happen. They say the pipe has the power of peace, of healing, of life.

Following the Buffalo Calf Woman come the warriors. Each wears a Sun Dance skirt from waist to ankles. Each enters the hoop, cradling his own pipe in his forearm. Then come the women; they too carry their own pipes. Inside the hoop, the sixty dancers stop at each of the four directions. Then they enter the covered resting place, placing their pipes against a forked stick altar before entering.

After each dance round, six or seven dancers pick up their pipes in an exchange ceremony. On the south side, they give it to someone picked from among the supporters, who then invites others to share it. By day's end, every pipe will have been exchanged and smoked by hundreds of people.

During most rounds, some dancers are pierced. When it is a dancer's turn, he lies on a buffalo-hide rug at the base of the sacred tree, while holy men make two parallel incisions to lift a finger-width strip of skin on each side of his chest or his back with a surgical scalpel. A round, sharpened piece of wood is thrust under the skin. No one cries out during the piercing.

The peg is fastened to the dancer's rope which is tied to the Sun Dance pole. Each dancer walks backwards as far as his rope allows and, leaning away from the pole, he dances until the skin breaks. That moment is one of liberation. The dancer, in triumph, circles the hoop joyfully. Some whose backs are pierced drag buffalo skulls behind them around the perimeter of the circle until the skin breaks. The moment of release is one of ecstasy.

I do not have difficulty with the ordeal. The Sacred Pole is a Tree of Life, as the Torah of the Jews is "a tree of life to those who hold fast to it," says the Talmud. Jews reminds themselves of this gift every morning at dawn. They bind leather straps on their arms and heads as a commitment that their hearts and minds must stay connected to this tree of life if they as a people are to survive. Indeed, the healing of the earth depends upon their doing this. The Lakotas' Sun Dance is remarkably similar in purpose and symbol.

During the evenings and early morning hours of the Sun Dance, everyone in the camp can participate in sweat ceremonies. The sweat lodges go long into the night, as long as there are people waiting. Like the Sun Dance and the pipe, they are sacred ceremonies. Inside the sweat lodge, the pipe is passed to each participant. Everyone holds it, smokes it, and gets a turn to speak.

At my turn, I sing a song in Hebrew and find myself joined by another voice! Here, in the middle of the eastern Oregon forest, at a sacred Indian ceremony, I am singing in Hebrew and with another member of my tribe! The power of this moment fills me with a sense of the spirit in this place. In the blackness, I am moved to tears. I am unashamed because I cannot be seen, but I feel naked before the spirit.

On the afternoon of the third day, Brave Buffalo calls me into the circle to receive a pipe in the exchange from one of the warriors. It is an honor to be called forth. As the young warrior approaches me with his pipe, he stops and whispers to the leader that he doesn't want to exchange it with me. I don't know whether he has picked someone else, or if he dislikes me or maybe white people in general. But I feel that he ought to be able to choose anyone he wants to support him during this ordeal. I am asked to step back and somebody else comes forward.

Brave Buffalo later tells me that what happened really isn't the way. You don't refuse to exchange your pipe if someone has been selected to come forward to receive it; it is in the exchange that one actually understands the meaning of the Sun Dance. When people share that pipe they fulfill the prophetic message of the coming together of all the peoples and colors of the four directions in a harmony of Spirit to perpetuate the earth and everything that lives on it.

I told myself I was not hurt by the warrior's rejection, but I was.

The next day I am called forward again. I would have been happy to stay back; I didn't want to be refused again. But if you're picked, you are expected to participate even if you don't feel ready to; someone else must feel you are and that's why you were picked. That degree of trust encourages one to get out of old conditioning and take a chance at spontaneity.

I step forward and, as only happens in the movies, I find myself opposite the same dancer who refused me the day before. This time he offers me his pipe. I appreciate what his choosing to approach me again says about him.

We stand not more than two feet apart and look at each other, but we don't speak. Four times we reach out to each other, and on the last time he gives me his sacred pipe. I smoke the pipe with others and tell them how pleased I am to have stepped forward and confronted my fear of rejection (my ego, my narcissism). When I return his pipe to him, we look at each other again, still silent.

That night I dream about my daughter and her boyfriend, a very nice guy, but not a member of my tribe. Because he didn't know my songs and dances, and I think he doesn't care, I've judged him badly. In my dream I see the two of them in some imminent danger. I rush to warn them of a disaster, but they can't seem to hear me. I am stopped by an invisible plastic shield that insulates them. I scream and bang on it, but they do not hear me. I am feeling more desperation and wake up with a start, sweating, my heart pounding.

In the predawn light I understand what I came to the Sun Dance to learn. That dancer judged me as unacceptable, for whatever reason. But he chose to come back to me. I judged the boyfriend, but I never came back to him, and now I was about to lose my daughter.

When the Sun Dance ends, the dancers emerge from the circle for the first time since they entered four days earlier. They greet the rest of us who are lined up outside. I shake hands and hold the dancer with whom I exchanged the pipe. Still, we don't speak.

That night at the celebration, I tell Brave Buffalo about my dream. I wonder aloud whether to seek out the dancer to share my insight and thank him. Brave Buffalo asks, "Why?

You only understand it as you understand it. How you see it is just the way it is for you. For him too it is as it is. The hope is that we try to see it in as many ways and as many times as we can."

So this is how I see it for now:

Once I was comfortable only with speaking words; I have since learned to sing, to pray, to touch. I reveal and I listen; I sometimes light candles and cedar. Whenever I used only one dimension in the healing process, I minimized my potential healing power. I had to feel my power to know it, and now I can't imagine it differently. There is a world beyond our own awareness.

The Sioux, the Cheyenne, the Assiniboin, the Blackfeet, and the Mandan were defeated by war and disease. The great buffalo were rendered nearly extinct; the people of the Plains were deprived of a way of life, but not of their spirit.

When Black Elk was an old man, he asked to be taken back to the Sacred Mountain where he first saw his vision. There he spoke to the Great Spirit, Wakan Tanka.

> Grandfather, with tears, I say to you that our nation's hoop is broken and scattered. This is not the center any longer. The sacred tree does not bloom here. Where you took me when I was young and taught me, here I stand now, as an old man, in sorrow and feeble voice. The tree is withered. If some little root still lives, may it leaf and bloom and fill with singing birds. May it bloom not for myself but for my people that they may once more go back to the sacred hoop and find the good Red Road, the Shielding Tree.

It is a tree of life to those who hold fast to it. Everyone needs a tree.

Kallah

After the Sun Dance sweat lodge ceremony, as we all mingled outside, a man approached me and thanked me for my song. He said he had thought about singing in Hebrew but wondered whether it was appropriate.

I repeated, as I had heard it, that as long as you had a language in which you prayed and a song that carried its message, it was always appropriate. At least you and the Creator understand the words, and the others will appreciate your efforts.

I thanked him too. In all my experience in Indian country, I told him, this was the first time anybody had ever joined me in singing in my own language. How moved I felt, indeed how awed, to be in this isolated, spiritual place and to find there a member of my tribe.

Aryeh turned out to be a rabbi. He came to the Sun Dance because here he could feel the spirit. He held feathers as he danced, and he brought his prayer shawl and phylacteries—those leather straps of devotion—to greet the morning sun.

Aryeh received his ordination from a New Age Hasidic rabbi, Reb Zalman Schacter. Reb Zalman was trained by the Lubavitch Hasidim in Brooklyn. In the fomenting 1960s he found a ready audience of young Jews who responded to his mystical worldview.

Reb Zalman at first went to Canada and later became a professor of Jewish Mysticism at Temple University and a teacher at the Reconstructionist Rabbinical College in Philadelphia. He is also "Rebbe in Residence" and founder of B'nai Or, the Followers of Light, a traditionally oriented Jewish community organized around the belief that all learning takes place within the context of a spiritual life and that one can expand old religious paradigms to find new ways to experience awe. Reb Zalman also ordains rabbis, which is a little bit controversial in the organized hierarchy of official learning.

Aryeh asked me to join him in morning prayers the following day. It had been a long time since I had greeted the sun in the company of another Jew. I joined him in my prayer shawl, the same one I wear in the tipi. Aryeh wore a prayer shawl of many colors such as I had never seen before.

In the morning, as we sang in Hebrew, Ivdu HaShem b'simcha, "Worship God with Joy," I heard in the distance the Sun Dancers entering the sacred circle and blowing their eagle-bone whistles. It is the first time I can remember greeting the dawn with tears.

Here in Indian country my heart again opened to an appreciation of the mystery. For a long time this part of me had cried to be filled, but I did not want to acknowledge this need Here, in the unassuming simplicity of the ceremonies, I felt a connection to a sense of the infinite and an appreciation of the spirit in the small things I had too long taken for granted

My wife is not moved in the ways I am at Indian spiritual gatherings. She yearned to touch that part of herself in a Jew ish environment and was frightened by my growing distance from it.

After our morning service, I asked Aryeh about the multicolored prayer shawl. He told me it was the result of a Reb Zalman vision, a dream about the biblical account of how God wrapped himself in a "cloak of light" before creating the universe. Zalman saw the shawl as having all the colors of the rainbow; he says he no longer sees things as just black or white.

As soon as I got home, I sent away to find out more about B'nai Or.

The following year, almost at the exact time of the previous year's Sun Dance, B'nai Or sponsored a Kallah or spiritual retreat. It would include a "vision quest." A rabbi, inspired by a Lakota spiritual leader with whom he studied, had translated an Indian worldview into a Jewish liturgical experience. We would meet as a tribe the evening before our quest and prepare ourselves to respond to God's challenge to Abraham and Sarah to reach beyond themselves in order to find their deepest selves. It was an offer I could not refuse, and it seemed made to order as a way for my wife, Elaine, and me to reexperience a Jewish spiritual rootedness.

We participated in workshops on future visioning and mask-making, dancing and praying from the inside. The vision quest was held on the Sabbath eve.

The evening before, sixty of us meet as a group. The Rebbe lights sage and passes it around in an abalone shell.

He talks about questing from a Jewish mystical perspective: how both concepts emphasize solitude, you go alone to seek enlightenment; how both require ritual cleansing and the use of objects and special garments to protect oneself from evil influences. Both acknowledge spirit messages and messengers. Both encourage altered states of consciousness through deprivation, fasting, and prayer, and in both there is the hope of receiving guidance through the spirit.

We sing the ancient chants, and each of us picks a card on which is written one word that is to serve as a meditation focus in tomorrow's silence. Mine says "knowingness."

Before dawn the following morning, we gather in an oak grove to recite the morning prayers. The Rebbe has picked selections from the liturgy that I had never heard: prayers about guardian spirits, animals, the earth, and the four directions.

The morning is shrouded in a misty fog. With the first light, some stand and wrap the leather straps of devotion to their arms and heads. In the distance, thunder rumbles while we chant, "The Earth, the Water, the Fire, the Air, Return Return Return." I feel again the tears at dawn.

The morning service breaks; it is now the time of silence and solitude. I wander silently, my prayer shawl draped on my shoulders. I stroll through a Catholic college campus with religious statuary everywhere and smile to think how Mother Cabrini would appreciate the scene. I smell a flower, and for a long, long time watch an inchworm slowly cross a leaf; it is a modern dancer.

Sitting on a playground swing, I think psychotherapy is a vision quest with the psychiatrist as guide to help facilitate the experience.

I walk up a hill and come upon the Rebbe in a tree. He is *in* the tree—not on a branch but sitting inside a cavelike hollow in its trunk. He sits totally enveloped by his prayer shawl.

"The Rebbe in a tree." The music of it, the clarity: "the Rebbe is in a tree." In every tree, a Rebbe, in every tree and in every thing. There is a spirit in all things.

When I come to the next tree, I wrap my arms around it. I feel it; I feel its aliveness; it hums. A bug crawls out of the tree, right under my nose, and I can feel its steps—it dances. I have never looked at a bug so closely.

Continuing my walk, I am caught by surprise again: here in the middle of Pennsylvania, right in the middle of an amphitheater, I have come upon a tipi. I discovered that I have wandered onto the grounds of a military academy that uses the tipi for some ceremonial occasion.

Today it's just standing there empty. I go inside and take out the cedar I brought with me knowing there would come a time to use it. I fill the tipi with its fragrance. A soft rain against the tipi's outside sounds like music on a canvas drum. I enshroud myself with my prayer shawl.

I am the Rebbe in this tree. Everyone of us a Rebbe. We are the language of the creative source and with all things we are as kin. Again I feel tears of unexplainable joy.

I remember my word: "knowingness." I don't "know" how I found this place but I know I want to experience it again. This is what I want to be, to accept things as I experience them and accept that there are things I will never "know."

This openness makes life's journey not only tolerable but allows us, again and again, to experience awe. Awe: that moment of insight into meaning other than ourselves, meaning in the small things that help us recognize the presence of the infinite.

A couple of weeks after the Kallah, I attended the Big Mountain Sun Dance. Sitting under the covered arbor day after day was a paralyzed woman in a wheelchair. She had use only of her fingers, just enough to move an electrical switch to control the movement of her chair. To get to the arbor, she had to be pushed along a rugged path. Once she arrived, she stayed all day.

On the afternoon of the third day, a warrior (himself crippled with a shriveled leg), was struggling to drag the skulls attached to the wooden pins in the flesh of his back. Already weak, he had twice circled the hoop. Friends and relatives entered the circle to stand behind him. Fanning him with feathers, they whispered encouragement.

In my heart, I wanted to step inside and be part of this group, but my feet would not move. (I don't know this man. What will others think?) My heart speaks, but my feet have a mind of their own.

The woman in the wheelchair asked somebody to push her into the circle. As a young man pushed her among those who followed the struggling Sun Dancer, she came to a complete stop directly in front of me—the wheels of the chair were sunk in six inches of sand. Had she stopped a foot in front of me or behind me I would have been spared the need to decide to step forward. My feet carried me, and while the other man pulled, I pushed her. Together we moved around the circle.

Here was a woman who was totally immobilized but whose heart, mind, and body followed the harmony of her truth. She knew she wanted to step in, so she did it. Yet I, who can move, needed her direct invitation to connect with my truth.

Sometimes it is the crippled who help us walk and the blind who help us see. What do I know? I know that had she not stopped directly in front of me, I would not have moved.

She stopped to help me move. In this small thing I sense the awesome presence of the mysterious.

Chapter 14

 BEAR BUTTE

In the fall of 1985 I addressed a conference of Indian hospital program directors on the subject of "Indian Perspectives on Healing." The conference was held in Rapid City, South Dakota, a place I had wanted to visit for a long time.

The Black Hills of South Dakota and Bear Butte are most sacred places for the Sioux, the Cheyenne, and all the tribes of the Plains. It was to this sacred mountain called Bear Butte that Red Cloud came for help and guidance before the so-called Red Cloud Wars. This is the place of Crazy Horse, Sitting Bull, and Black Elk; and it is here that the Cheyenne received the four sacred arrows that still sustain the spiritual life of their people.

Here also friends whom I call relatives have come on their own vision quests, to spend up to four days and nights on the peak seeking enlightenment. Bear Butte is a place of spiritual reflection, a place to seek direction, to look at what purpose you serve—a place of decision.

I wanted to experience this sacred place, but I did not anticipate that this visit would add this closing chapter to my years in Indian country, a step in my seeking to become a healer, in my own vision quest.

Before my trip to Bear Butte I visited the Sioux Indian Museum in downtown "Rapid." The museum was offering items for sale as part of a building fund drive. On one table I spotted a seventy-five-year-old elaborately beaded and quilled Sioux tobacco pouch. I could not resist. With the pouch came a small pipe. I also bought rattle used by the Yuwipi medicine men in the healing ceremonies of the Sioux.

As I drove toward Bear Butte, I thought, why not carry the sacred instruments to the peak? It was a unique chance to rededicate them to the purpose for which they were intended. I wanted to accept them in a good way, to say that I would keep them and use them the best way I knew how, and to cleanse them and me from whatever negative influences might interfere with such a recommitment. I felt good about the decision as I drove toward Bear Butte.

Bear Butte is a sacred place, and it's also a state park open to everyone. It has a ranger station, a small museum, marked trails, and lookout platforms; at its base live a small herd of buffalo. The butte rises like a volcanic marble two thousand feet above the flat plains. It has served as a landmark to pioneers and prospectors, to the cavalry and Custer.

On this drizzly day with clouds hanging low in the sky not many people were at the park. The ranger station was closed. I parked in the lot at the trail base, took a backpack from the trunk of my car, and laid the pipe and pouch on top of it. As I locked the car a young woman approached me.

Seeing the instruments she asked if I was going to load my pipe and pray on the sacred peak. I said I was going to dedicate my instruments there. Tearfully she told me that her grandmother had died the previous day. She and her relatives had come today to pray for her journey. Would I remember her in my prayers? she asked. I felt honored to do so.

She spoke of her grandmother, and I listened. It felt good to communicate this way. There were no questions about pedigree, blood, or tribe, just a shared appreciation of the power of the instruments and the sacramental quality of the place.

I packed the things and jauntily started walking toward the sweat lodges at the volcano's base. Feeling cheerful, happy with my purchase, glad to be in this place, gratified by the stranger's confidence, I sauntered up the path. As I approached the grounds, I was stopped cold by a rattling sound. Eighteen inches in front of me a rattlesnake was coiled into striking position, its head flattened and rattle humming. I moved back gingerly. I had never been so close to a rattler in the wild. I started talking to it.

"Be cool. I know you were here first, this is your place. I'm moving back. Be cool." Then, with a flush of societal embarrassment, I looked around to see if anyone was watching me talk to a snake.

Indians have a special thing about snakes. They see them as messengers that move like lightning. Pay attention when these animal brothers move, their entire beings are in contact with the Earth; they can hear the heartbeat of the Earth Mother with their whole body. We are in contact with it only with our feet.

It is the animals who tell us of forthcoming earthquakes, not machines or people. Snakes carry a message about the place where we live: if you don't treat this place carefully, if you march too merrily, if you don't take this place and your purpose on it seriously, something bad will happen. I got the message: don't step lightly. Be serious about what you're here for, what you are about to do, how others have come here before you. This is a sacred place. Don't get captivated by your ego.

I appreciated the reminder; I needed it. I approached the sweat lodge grounds with a wholly different kind of bounce.

Two sweat-lodge frames of willow had been erected. All around them trees were covered with ribbons, scarves, tobacco-filled cloth pouches in the colors of the four directions; even the bushes had the red, yellow, white, and black ties on their branches. Feathers tied to prayer sticks were implanted in front of the lodge frames. The colors fluttered everywhere. You could feel them, like living ornaments blowing wishes.

I shivered with the power of the place and felt the presence of a hundred years of initiates who had come here to prepare for the quest. I touched the pipe rack, the altar, the prayer stick, then tied my own offerings. I continued climbing the path and watched the Great Plains stretch out below. I could see circling wagons and hear screaming warriors. I could see the earth black with buffalo and feel it move with their stampeding. The place was filled with the energy of imagination.

On the hike up the well-traveled trail of Bear Butte I could see colored cloth prayer offerings everywhere, some with tiny items tied in them. In some trees stones are embedded, placed there years before by the faithful.

And paths branching from the main trail are blocked by signs that say: "Indians Praying: Do Not Disturb." How wonderful! We need such signs in every state park, in every forest, and on every waterway. It changes your whole way of looking at a place if you know people are praying there, that the Earth is the cathedral. It says more about why we should respect the Earth than "Don't Step on the Grass," "Keep Out," or "Do Not Litter."

Indians Praying. Do Not Disturb.

At the peak, a marker on a tree cautions hikers not to continue. These are the vision quest grounds.

I feel my hands tingling. The trees are covered with prayer scarves. On both sides of the slopes, as far as my eye can see, rectangles of at least four square feet are formed by strings connected to four trees. The strings are dotted with tiny cloth bundles filled with tobacco and flesh offerings.

During the quest one of these enclosures becomes the center of all things. Here the vision quester sits for days, without eating. A doorway is created by placing two pieces of sage over one of the strings; the quester can enter and exit the space through this "door"; When he or she is inside, the sage is removed.

Here a quester might touch the spark of light that we call insight.

How we need such sacramental places. They don't have to be on a mountaintop or in a temple. Each of us can find this place on our own path, a place that speaks to us in a special way. We make it sacred by separating it from the ordinary world by physical markings or by our attitude. We need to find and recognize the sacred places on our path, to go back to them for sustenance, for centering.

I find an enclosed rectangle nestled into the western slope. I will stay for a while. I leave my pack outside, collect two forked sticks and a cross bar. In the sacred place I make a pipe rack and rest my instruments on it. I light some cedar I brought from Arizona.

I pray. Prayer is whenever you allow your tongue and lips to move synchronously with your heart without first processing your feelings through your head.

The smoke's fragrance bathes me; it separates this place from the ordinary. It removes the lampshades that keep me from appreciating my own light.

I pray about friends, family, ancestors, animals, and the dead grandmother. I pray about my future. In the drizzle, I offer the pipe. My life breath is illuminated in smoke; it seems to make the raindrops stop in midair.

As I sit I wonder how I got here. By what path did I come to this point in my life, in my work?

I think, on the mountain, that in my work as a psychiatrist I am another guide for people seeking vision. I am a guide who helps people process life's experience and find the message within about who we are, what our purposes are, what our paths are. What I do is just another ritualized vision quest. My patients invest my workplace and my ceremony with power; if they believe in my language, in what I know, then they can receive what I have to say to them.

Society has endowed psychiatry with the mantle of legitimacy as the best way to help us make sense of our history. But there are so many ways that can allow us a glimpse into meaning. The important thing is to seek a vision on your path and with someone you trust, someone who speaks your language, who appreciates your dance.

If you choose to make the journey, you will always find guides.

On my way down from the top of Bear Butte I picked up some stones to put in my medicine bundle. I would share and thereby remember some of the healing of this place.

Weeks later I again saw the snake—in a dream. Coiled and rattling, it now spoke to me, but I couldn't hear it. I saw the tongue darting but I couldn't hear the words.

Again the snake. It is these seemingly small events that make up the legends of our lives.

I understand now. It is not what the snake says that is important, but what the snake is. It is my power animal, my reminder. I hear it saying, "You are the messenger. Tell the story before the earth quakes."

So this is the story. I've shared the steps that I learned the best way I know how. I hope they help you to hear your music.

People

PHOTOGRAPHY

A GUIDE TO TAKING BETTER PICTURES

Michael Coyne

LONELY PLANET OFFICES

Australia
Head Office
Locked Bag 1, Footscray, Victoria 3011
☎ 03 8379 8000, fax 03 8379 8111
talk2us@lonelyplanet.com.au

UK
72–82 Rosebery Ave,
Clerkenwell, London EC1R 4RW
☎ 020 7841 9000, fax 020 7841 9001
go@lonelyplanet.co.uk

USA
150 Linden St, Oakland, CA 94607
☎ 510 893 8555, toll free 800 275 8555
fax 510 893 8572, info@lonelyplanet.com

People Photography: A Guide to Taking Better Pictures

1st edition May 2005
ISBN 1 74059 541 6

Published by Lonely Planet Publications Pty Ltd
ABN 36 005 607 983

text © Lonely Planet 2005
photographs © Michael Coyne 2005

Cover photograph: Young girl in traditional costume, Melaka, Malaysia

 Many of the images in this guide are available for licensing from
Lonely Planet Images: www.lonelyplanetimages.com.

Printed through The Bookmaker International Ltd.
Printed in China

CONTENTS

THE AUTHOR

Michael Coyne, when at home, lives in Melbourne, Australia. As an award-winning professional photographer, most of his time is spent travelling the world photographing people. His first photographs were taken with a borrowed Kodak Box Brownie when he was 11 years old and travelling with his parents through the Panama Canal. These first pictures were travel photographs of people.

His professional career began when he took a job with the *Australian* newspaper in Melbourne. In the decades since, he has travelled to every corner of the globe. He has worked on assignments for, and his photographs have appeared in, magazines and newspapers such as *National Geographic, Newsweek, Time, Life, Smithsonian, Condé Nast Traveler, Travel Holiday, Reader's Digest, German Geo,* the *Independent and* the *Observer.* Seven books of his photographs have been published. He has had a large number of exhibitions and his photographs are in collections in Washington, DC; New York; San Francisco; Sydney; Melbourne; London and Rome. Michael lectures on photography and has given photography workshops in Australia and New Zealand, Asia, Africa and Central America.

From the Author

Writing this book has given me a wonderful opportunity to rethink and to share the knowledge and skills learnt in a lifetime of photography. I have been fortunate to be paid for what I love doing the most: travelling the world and photographing people in places which always seem new, even if I've been there many times before. Every time I return, the light is different and there are new people to portray. The day I lose my sense of wonder about the inexhaustible variety of people on this planet is the day I shall quit photography. That day, I suspect, will never come.

I'm a people photographer. I'm entranced when I listen to people's stories and share their lives and experiences. I've drunk tea with nomads in Iran, eaten mealie with tribespeople in Africa and danced the tango with gauchos in Argentina. Travelling, and photographing and meeting people, is all I've ever wanted to do.

My colleagues, assistants and collaborators are far too many to thank, especially because the chief collaborators in any good photograph are often the people being photographed. So my first thanks must go to the many thousands of people who have permitted me to photograph them. They have welcomed me into their lives, no matter how fleeting and yet long-lasting the moment. I would also like to thank Rob Gale, Sue and Neil Jackson, Steve Bent, Alfred Wong, Jean Murdoch, Catherine Coyne, Greg Tinkler, Naomi Stevenson, James Marshall, Roger Garwood, Martin Brooke, Eric Soh, Roger Stewart of CPL and Sim Siang Hock, John Swainston and Julie Matroski of Nikon. My gratitude also goes to Graham Pitts, an old friend who has been an invaluable reader and advisor on the text. Most especially my thanks go to Anne, my wife, for her advice and patience and for taking the picture of me on the back cover. Lonely Planet commissioned and guided this book to publication. So, thank you Richard I'Anson of Lonely Planet. It has been a great experience.

THIS BOOK

From the Publisher

This book was produced in Lonely Planet's Melbourne office. It was commissioned by Laetitia Clapton and series editor Richard I'Anson. Bridget Blair managed the project with assistance from Jo Vraca and Andrew Weatherill. Brigitte Barta and Janet Austin edited. The book was designed by Brendan Dempsey and laid out by Steven Cann. Radek Wojcik did the cover artwork and Ryan Evans, Gerard Walker and Claire Gibson managed preparation of the images.

Using this Book

People Photography gives you the information you need to progress from taking basic shots that record the people you meet on your travels to capturing great photographs that evoke personality, lifestyle, background and environment. It aims to show you how to make the most of the equipment you use, from compact point-and-shoot cameras to advanced SLRs, whether you capture your images on film or digitally. It also suggests ways to approach and communicate with your subjects, how to compose better images, how to make the light work for you and how to make every photo opportunity count. Above all, it aims to make photographing people easier. The first rule of photography is simple: enjoy it. The second rule is equally enjoyable: keep it simple.

The Author's Approach

For me, the best photo assignments are a journey into the world of people. They might be dancers in Bali, cowboys in Patagonia, tribesmen in New Guinea or jugglers in Germany. I try to take photographs that celebrate human individuality and reflect the atmosphere and the ambience generated by people. Ideally, everything in the photograph is about the subject and nothing else.

Yet I have to acknowledge that every photograph reveals something, however minimal, about the photographer. For every photograph is the result of an array of creative but personal decisions about subject, camera format, lens, film type and speed, exposure, viewpoint and composition. Sometimes these decisions may have been wrong. At others time they were right. But they all add up to what I suppose is called my 'style'.

My style is reflected in my choice of equipment when working on personal projects, such as books or exhibitions. When I'm travelling my preferred system on such projects is:

▶ a 15-year-old Nikon FM2 camera body

▶ 20mm f2.8, 35mm f2 and 85mm f2 lenses

It's quick and easy to work with for candid and street photography and I feel the camera and lens combination is unobtrusive, allowing me to go virtually unnoticed. Typically, I have one of the three lenses on the camera body and the other two in my jacket pockets.

My travel camera bag is a Tamrac. It fits comfortably in a plane locker and holds all my basic gear. The bag looks like a backpack and to a possible thief doesn't look worth stealing.

On assignments I carry a lot more equipment, which I vary depending on the subject matter and location. I still shoot a lot of assignments on film but more and more I'm being asked by my clients to shoot digitally. Typically I'll pack:

- two Nikon F100 camera bodies for film
- a Nikon FM2 camera body for film
- two Nikon D100 camera bodies for digital capture
- three Nikon zoom lenses: a 17-35mm f2.8, a 35-70mm f2.8 and an 80-200mm f2.8
- five Nikkor fixed focal-length lenses: a 20mm f2.8, a 24mm f2, a 35mm f2, an 85mm f2 and a 300mm f4.5 or 300mm f2.8
- a Nikon SB25 Speedlight
- a Nikon SB-80DX Speedlight
- two Quantum battery packs
- a Minolta flash meter
- a Gitzo tripod with a ball head
- a monopod
- a table-top tripod
- silver foil (for use as a reflector)
- a Tamrac camera bag (big enough for my standard outfit and fits comfortably in a plane locker)
- a Zero Halliburton case (for locking up spare equipment left in the hotel room).

All the lenses have Nikon L1BC filters to protect the front element from dust and scratches. When I'm shooting colour transparency film and I want to add a little extra warmth to skin tones, I use a Nikon 81A, 81B or 81C warming filter.

The other accessories I usually have in my case are: reflectors, colour gels, spare AA batteries, lens-cleaning cloth, lens cleaner tissues, blower brush, film-leader retriever, two cable releases, model-release forms, notebook, labels to identify film, gaffer tape, marker pen, small flashlight, Blu-tack, Swiss Army knife, pliers, sun cream, small towel, small medical kit and plastic zip bags for carrying film as well as for keeping cameras and lenses dry.

When walking the streets on assignment, I don't carry all of this equipment. Most of it is left back at the hotel for when it's needed. But what I do carry with me are two camera bodies and two zoom lenses, a 17-35mm lens and either a 35-70mm lens or an 80-200mm lens, depending on the type of assignment and location.

Over the years I've used many different films, including Kodachrome 25, 64 and 200. Currently, I use Fujichrome Sensia II RA 100 or Ektachrome E100GX 100, depending on the light and subject and the result I require. In low light I use Ektachrome E200 and occasionally push it one or two stops. If colour negative is required I use either Fujicolor NPS 160 or Fujicolor NPH 400. For black-and-white images I shoot with Kodak T-Max rated at 100 or 400 ISO.

On location I always wear shirts with long sleeves and extra pockets. I like to be protected from the sun, and the extra pockets come in handy for film, memory cards, pens and notes.

Photo Captions

The photographs in this book illustrate many different ways of photographing people, and were taken in a wide range of circumstances. The captions explain some of the contexts, intentions and technical details – hopefully this will help your own understanding of what is photographically possible at various times and places. They include information about:

- camera, lens and film type (though please note that some films are no longer available and that the name of the film changes from country to country)
- shutter speed and aperture, if known
- tripod, filters and flash, if used.

INTRODUCTION

People are by far the most popular subject for photography, as they endlessly charm, entertain and fascinate. And photographing people is the most accessible and popular form of art. Indeed the price of the sort of camera you need to take a great photograph is now more affordable than it has ever been. However, photography's popularity is not solely due to accessibility. Humans seem to possess an ageless desire to capture significant images of others and the places in which they live. Cave dwellers of more than 50 thousand years ago came back from their nomadic hunts to paint on cave walls the things they had witnessed. Since the dawn of photography, the same desire to share an experience has led modern travellers to bring back a pictorial record of places and, especially, the people they've encountered when travelling.

A similar human need for self-expression has produced thousands of great painted portraits, many of which have stood the test of time and are found in galleries around the world. They can provide much inspiration to a photographer regarding composition, framing, colour and choice of subject. It's also intriguing to see how painting has changed since the advent of photography and how much modern painters have learnt from photographers. The hours within a day unsuitable for photography are never wasted by a visit to an art gallery. It might well contain the work of other photographers as well as painted portraits. In any case, masterworks of portraiture endlessly fascinate because they both capture and transcend the concept the artist and photographer originally envisaged.

For the people photographer the most important thing is the ability to see the world and its people as never before; to see the potential in every face and figure, every setting and every possible option of matching person and setting; to see vivid colours and all the subtle tones between black and white that are part of everyday life. Every photograph you take increases your ability to see people with additional insight and adds to your appreciation of ever-present beauty. This is often achieved by photographing people in their own environment – the places where they work, play or pray.

Great people photographs reveal an amazing amount about the subject's personality and character. They provide insights into inner emotions and, often, the world inhabited by the subject. As photographer Alfred Eisenstaedt said, 'The camera lets you see ordinary people in extraordinary ways'.

Whether a photograph is of an individual or a group of people, fills the frame with someone's face or includes the environment as an integral part of the composition, a really good people picture catches your first glance and then holds you, for it has many levels of meaning. You can look at such photos again and again, discovering something new and different every time. They reveal many external characteristics about the subject such as gender, age and ethnicity, but they also go beyond the surface by providing insights into a person's character, occupation, hobbies, diet, religion, culture, social position, emotions, mood, spirit and the way they see themselves.

Monk in front of painting, Siem Riep, Cambodia

◄ 35mm SLR, 35mm lens, 1/60 f2, Ektachrome E100G

PEOPLE IN COLOUR

Good colour images are created through the conscious use of particular hues to strengthen or enhance the balance of the image. A picture of someone can be bland or exciting simply because of the colours you choose to exclude or include, and including all colours without first pausing to think of the consequences can be the photographic equivalent of being colour-blind.

Colour is emotionally evocative. We respond with different feelings to blue skies, orange sunsets, green forests or a yellow swathe of corn in a field. Similarly, too, we all react consciously or subconsciously to the hues and colours of the clothes people wear. People also react to the palette of colours you use in the foreground or background when the environment is part of your picture.

Photographer Rob Gale believes 'Colours are evocative of time, place and people; they play a big part in how vividly we perceive and remember other human beings. When we travel we see how differently people around the world express themselves through their use of colour. The colours that we see used in a city like Sydney are very different to colours that we see in Kathmandu, which are different again to the colours people use in Las Vegas or Beijing.'

Three women in saris, Samode, India

The golden field of grain, lit by the early-morning light, wonderfully matches the yellow of the women's saris. The bright red and greens they wear provide contrast. Sometimes it pays to seek out bright colours but make sure they don't merge into similar or matching colours in the environment.

▲ 35mm SLR, 35mm lens, 1/250 f5.6, Ektachrome E100G

**Shepherd boy,
Adjibar, Ethiopia**

The afternoon fog on a hilltop
swirls around the boy and his
herd, creating soft and muted
colours. If you know the full
capabilities of your equipment
it's possible to photograph
beautiful colours in any sort of
weather.

◀ 35mm SLR, 35mm lens, 1/125 f4,
Sensia 100

PEOPLE IN BLACK & WHITE

The potential for successful black-and-white pictures of people should not be overlooked. Black-and-white images can show human shapes, skin textures, subtle tones and shades of photographic meaning at times when colour would be a distraction. The tonal balance between a rich deep black and a clear clean white can embody or powerfully suggest a wide range of feelings and emotions. To learn to see in black and white, start to look for form, content and emotion.

There are times when shooting in black and white offers distinct advantages over colour. For example, it's possible to achieve great images in low or bad light. Additionally, if you're shooting on film, you don't have to take the effect of the colour of artificial lighting into consideration. This, in turn, allows for more spontaneous and candid photography in artificially lit settings. One of the most compelling reasons for shooting in black and white is that without the constraints and considerations of colour you have the freedom to concentrate on the essential qualities of the person you are seeking to portray.

Fishermen on beach, Dili, East Timor

It's critically important to study the way light falls on people when photographing in black and white. One of these fishermen was sitting down. Then he suddenly stood up, rested his hand on his knee, and everything seemed to fall into place. Because of the direction of the sun I was able to use light and shade in a graphically balanced image.

▶ 35mm SLR, 35mm lens, 1/500 f8, Tri-X 400

Early morning smoke haze, Dili, East Timor

The silhouette of the man walking towards the smoke of a small fire might seem relatively insignificant. However, if you use the tip of your finger to cover his silhouetted figure, you will see that without him the picture is flat and featureless.

◀ 35mm SLR, 80-200mm lens at 200mm, 1/500 f8, Tri-X 400

**Playmates,
Dili, East Timor**

This picture would not
have worked as well
in colour. The clashing
bright colours of the boy's
shirt and shorts would
have been a distraction.
Black-and-white photog-
raphy helps you to focus
your attention on the key
elements of an image – in
this case the boy's face and
the dog.

◀ 35mm SLR, 35mm lens,
1/250 f5.6, Tri-X 400

It's also much easier to set yourself up to develop and print black-and-white film than it is to process and print colour negative or transparency film. If you shoot in black and white, consider processing your own film and making your own prints, for then you will be in complete control of the entire photographic process, from capture to print. You can print the photo as light or as dark as you wish. You can add in tone, shade and light. This is not possible to the same extent with colour film because of the need to outsource the processing.

Creating your own darkroom can be a surprisingly inexpensive process. It need not be permanent, and a bathroom is ideal due to the ready supply of water. You'll need to cover up the windows with black cloth or black plastic. Any leaks or spaces around the door through which light can leak should be taped over with black tape. (Black plastic and tape are usually available from your local hardware supplier.) Also ensure you have adequate shelf space for the enlarger, timer, papers, trays and chemicals. See the Further Reading section on p150 for books that contain sections on building your own darkroom.

**Early-morning exercise,
Hong Kong, China**

Almost all digital cameras shoot only in colour. But colour can often be distracting. I converted this image to black and white in Photoshop, which served to reduce the dominance of the background.

◀ DSLR, 35-70mm lens at 58mm, 1/200 f8, 400 ISO, 3008 x 2000, RAW

PART ONE:

The earliest photographers had to carry an enormous load of equipment and film when travelling. Even rudimentary portraits of people required heavy plate cameras, tripods, hoods, developing equipment and a host of devices. It was a very slow process. The subjects sat motionless, their head held by clamps, for anywhere between 15 to 25 seconds. Of course, this is no longer necessary. A photograph can now be taken in a thousandth of a second and seen instantly on a liquid-crystal display (LCD) screen on the back of a digital camera. Everything is much lighter and quicker now.

But some things don't change. There is an old maxim amongst photographers which says that if you're thinking about your equipment when taking a picture, you're not taking a good picture. So, practise with your equipment until it seems part of your body and mind. Practise working with it long before you leave home. There are few things worse than missing a potentially great picture because you don't yet understand your equipment well enough.

EQUIPMENT & FILM

A Chinese Opera performer, Singapore

◀ DSLR, 80-200mm lens at 135mm, 1/500 f3.2, 800 ISO, 3008 x 2000, RAW

EQUIPMENT

Your choice of equipment depends on three things: what you wish to achieve, what is comfortable and what is affordable. A basic point-and-shoot compact camera might be adequate to take quick snaps of the people you meet but the likelihood of achieving pictures of high quality greatly increases if you take along a single lens reflex (SLR) camera (either film or digital) with carefully selected lenses and accessories to suit your photographic goals.

Remember too that you have to carry the equipment on your journey so don't overburden yourself. The following system is very good and can be carried comfortably in a small camera bag:

▸ an SLR camera body (digital or film)
▸ a 24-80mm zoom lens
▸ an 80-200mm zoom lens
▸ a shoe-mount flash, preferably with a tilting head

Maori Worker, Awatoto, New Zealand

Sometimes a picture of a person can be more powerful and revealing when you photograph them from behind. This man had been loading bags onto a train and stopped for a break. Everything seemed to be balanced such as the dust on his head, the tattoos, his muscles and the straps on his back which complemented the straps on the train. Even if you photograph somebody from behind there is chance that they maybe recognised. If you have intentions of selling the image for commercial use get them to sign a model release.

▲ 35mm SLR, 85mm lens, 1/125 f5.6, Ektachrome E100VS

Women at Deepavali, Singapore

Deepavali is also known as the festival of lights because Hindus light oil lamps in their homes to thank the gods for peace, happiness and wealth. Women bath in oil and then pray at the temple wearing bright new clothes bought specially for the celebration. I stood behind a barrier which separated men from women, but I was still close enough to be able to use a wide-angle lens which captured the colour and vibrancy of the occasion.

◀ 35mm SLR, 20mm lens, 1/125 f11, Ektachrome E100GX

Man praying in a mosque, Singapore

Equipment as basic as a Nikon FM2 camera body and a 20mm lens can result in very rewarding images. The equipment was unobtrusive, simple and easy to work with. Note how the composition in the picture below is much more balanced with the inclusion of the man in the upper left of the image. In all three images the shadows play a very significant part. See how they either lead your eye to or from the man praying.

⬆ 35mm SLR, 20mm lens, 1/15 f4, Ektachrome E100G

🔺 35mm SLR, 20mm lens, 1/15 f4, Ektachrome E100G

◀ 35mm SLR, 20mm lens, 1/30 f4, Ektachrome E100G

CAMERAS

You can photograph people with any camera (film or digital). A simple point-and-shoot compact, a sophisticated SLR camera, a more specialist rangefinder camera and a cheap but exotic Holga all have their advantages and disadvantages. We'll focus primarily on the SLR camera and the lenses and accessories that are ideal for photographing people on the road.

SLR Cameras

If you're serious about capturing great pictures while you're on the road, a 35mm film or digital SLR (preferably one that allows you to manually override all of the automatic features) is the most suitable all-round camera for photographing people in the greatest variety of circumstances, situations and settings.

ADVANTAGES

▸ permits accurate compositions because the subject is viewed through the lens
▸ accepts a great variety of interchangeable lenses and accessories
▸ usually has a built-in flash, which allows you to balance the lighting and obtain pleasing portraits indoors and outdoors

DISADVANTAGES

▸ zoom lenses can be bulky and heavy
▸ the viewfinder blacks out for a split second when the shutter is pressed, so the photographer's view of the subject's movement or expression is interrupted at the instant the image is recorded

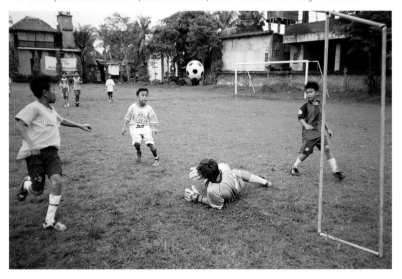

Soccer players, Ubud, Bali, Indonesia
It is possible to shoot good action pictures with a compact camera if you can get close and fill the frame with the people participating. I positioned myself about 3m from the players and followed the soccer ball through the viewfinder of the camera until the moment was right.

▲ 35mm compact, NPH 400

Water festival, Tampaksiring, Bali, Indonesia

The impact of this image, taken with a basic point-and-shoot compact camera, depends to a great extent on filling the frame with the subjects.

▲ 35mm compact, NPH 400

Balinese worshipping at a festival, Tampaksiring, Bali, Indonesia

Compact cameras are typically light, simple and easy to use. But this doesn't mean you just point the camera and hope. This picture doesn't have a point of focus, so the viewer's eye doesn't know where to go. The picture would have had more impact if it had been shot from the front, focussed on a section of the crowd or concentrated on one person.

▲ 35mm compact, NPH 400

Man with mannequin heads, Hong Kong, China

Many digital compact cameras take time to boot up, so make sure your camera is ready to go before approaching your subject. Fortunately, this shopkeeper remained in the position that attracted my attention while I waited for the camera to come to life.

▲ Compact digital, 2304 x 1704, fine JPEG

Hong Kong skyline, China

Compact digital cameras can capture great depth of field and sharpness if used when the light is optimal. In this picture you can see the details in the photographs in the foreground and the buildings all the way across the channel.

▲ Compact digital, 2304 x 1704, fine JPEG

OTHER CAMERAS

Compact Cameras

Compact film and digital cameras have basic settings and a non-interchangeable lens, and are intended primarily for taking snapshots. They often include a built-in flash, auto-focus and zoom lens. For people photography, it's best to choose a camera with a zoom lens which goes from standard to telephoto, rather than a wide-angle zoom lens.

ADVANTAGES

‣ a good camera with which to begin photographing people as it is so simple to use
‣ ideal for getting an instant record of people on your trip
‣ great for taking photos with a minimum of fuss, as people feel less threatened by small and innocuous equipment
‣ fully automatic, so you can take a series of pictures efficiently
‣ perfect if you want to travel light, as it can be carried in a pocket or handbag

DISADVANTAGES

‣ you can't get in very close to people because the minimum focussing distance is often around 1m
‣ limits the possibility of making large-size prints due to the lack of lens quality
‣ shutter speeds are sometimes slow, so it's not always possible to capture moving subjects
‣ when photographing people in low light, the flash will take over and destroy the natural light
‣ subjects are seen through a separate viewfinder and not the lens, so accurate framing is limited

Holga 120 Point-and-Shoot Cameras

A Holga is a cheap, medium-format, plastic film camera made in China. The shutter speed is set at approximately 1/100 of a second. There are two aperture settings: f11 for sunlight and f8 for cloudy or overcast days. It takes medium-format 120 roll film. Black-and-white or colour negative films provide the best results because of the unpredictability of the exposure. Holgas are becoming increasingly popular with people photographers, though they're still regarded by some as a mere toy. Depending on how it is used, it can be a plaything or a means of innovation. However, note that it is often expensive to get 120 film processed and that this is mainly done by professional labs.

ADVANTAGES

‣ light and extremely cheap (starting at US$30), so you can carry one as an extra camera and experiment with it
‣ good for vignetting, with the light brightest at the centre of the photograph and darker at the edges and corners; this allows you to photograph people so they look ethereal, otherworldly or from a different era
‣ no two Holgas are the same and they can provide unexpectedly wonderful and unusual photographs
‣ they are a great deal of fun

DISADVANTAGES

‣ it's necessary to shoot lots of film to guarantee you'll get a good result
‣ only works in reasonably good lighting, so you're limited to photographing people in bright light or, in the shade, using very fast film
‣ the minimum focussing distance is about 3 to 4.5 feet so it's not satisfactory for close-up portraits
‣ to stop the light leaking into the camera and destroying the film it's necessary to stick gaffer tape around the lens and back of the camera

⬍ Chicken boy, Dili, East Timor

⬏ Going to the market, Aileu, East Timor

▸ Young man, Dili, East Timor

East Timor is an island with a long history, and these pictures seem timeless, as if they could have been taken at any time since the advent of photography. To achieve this look I used a plastic pinhole-type point-and-shoot camera called a Holga. The film fogs around the edges, giving a vignette effect.

All images Holga 120, TRI-X 400

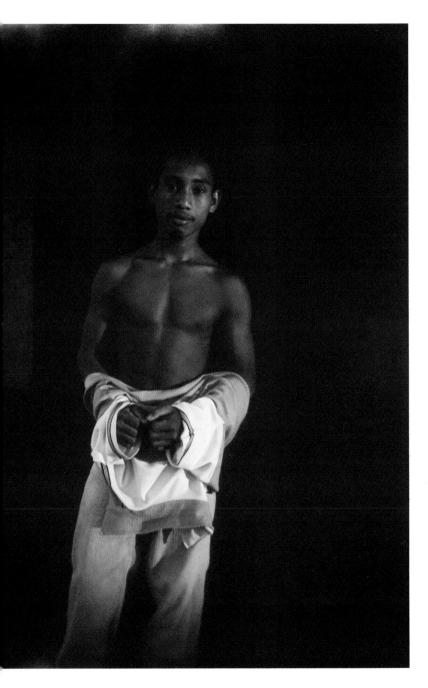

Rangefinders

The 35mm film and digital rangefinder cameras sit between compacts and SLRs in terms of size and features but are considerably more expensive than compacts. They're very popular with street photographers.

ADVANTAGES

‣ fast to work with when shooting candid pictures

‣ has a very quiet shutter so is great for photographing in theatres, churches, synagogues, mosques and other places of worship

‣ easy to focus in low light, so gives more opportunities to photograph people in covered areas such as markets

‣ the precision viewfinder allows you to see your subject at the exact moment you press the shutter

DISADVANTAGES

‣ no zoom lenses, so you will need to compose your pictures by physically moving or by changing the lens

‣ only a limited selection of telephoto lenses are available

‣ the flash synchronisation is 1/50 of a second, so it's not always possible to use the camera for fill-in flash when taking portraits

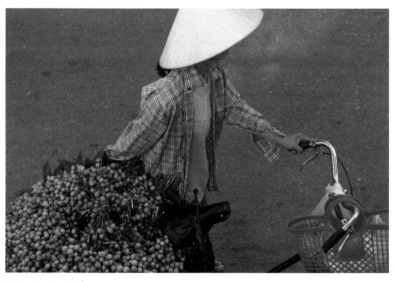

Market Day, Hanoi, Vietnam

People were moving along the road to the market with baskets and bags full of colourful produce. The background was a series of old rusty iron gates and walls which would have been distracting in my picture. So I climbed onto a wall and pointed the camera down which meant I could use the neutral colour of the road as a background. With a short zoom lens, 35 – 70mm attached to the camera I followed this woman in a panning motion and fired the shutter at the moment she was level with me.

▲ DSLR, 35-70mm lens at 70mm, 1/250 f5.6, 200 ISO, 3008 x 2000, RAW

LENSES FOR SLR CAMERAS

The ability to interchange lenses is one of the most persuasive reasons to buy a film or digital SLR. You can photograph people with any lens but some are better suited to certain subjects.

Standard Lenses

Standard lenses have focal lengths of 50mm or 55mm, with an angle of view that is close to what the eye sees, and they create images that are undistorted and natural. They're well suited for photographing small groups of people and general scenes at festivals and other public gatherings.

Telephoto Lenses

Medium telephotos range from 70mm to 105mm and make excellent portrait lenses. They give a pleasing perspective to the face and let you fill the frame with a head-and-shoulder composition without being in the face of your subject. Lenses of 135mm to 250mm focal length are ideal for picking faces out of a crowd. They also allow the frame to be filled when it's impossible to move in close to your subject, such as at sporting events or festivals.

Zoom Lenses

Zooms are extremely popular and the ideal choice for the travelling people photographer. They are very versatile, allowing you to shoot environmental portraits and close-ups with a single lens. They also allow various framing possibilities from a fixed position, including the ability to hold moving people in frame without having to move with them. If you only want to carry one lens, a 28-80mm is ideal for photographing people in a variety of situations.

Wide-Angle Lenses

These 28mm to 35mm wide-angle lenses allow you to capture more of your subject's environment than is possible with a standard (50mm to 55mm) lens. Unless you are looking for an unusual angle it is better not to have people standing at the edge of the frame, as they will be distorted (though not as greatly as they will be if you use a super wide-angle lens). Both wide-angle and super wide-angle lenses distort features if the subject is too close to the lens.

Stockman on horse, Mount Isa, Australia

This silhouette was shot with a semi-fisheye lens. This achieved a slight curve at the edges, helping to convey the sense of apparently limitless outback space.

◀ 35mm SLR, 15mm lens, 1/60 f4, Kodachrome 64

Super Wide-Angle Lenses

The super wide-angle lens group includes 20mm and 24mm lenses. They produce images that have a distinctly wide-angle perspective and are particularly suited to taking environmental portraits, especially where space is tight. They allow you to get close to your subject to create a sense of involvement in the picture while including the location as well.

Woman with red fan, Singapore

These t'ai chi exercises were shot with an 80-200mm zoom lens on a tripod. The first image was shot with a fast shutter speed and is very sharp but has a shallow depth of field. In the second image, shot with a medium shutter speed, there is slight blur of hand movement to help capture the graceful exercise. In the third image, shot with a slow shutter speed, zooming in with the lens creates an even more effective sense of movement.

◀ DSLR, 80-200mm lens at 200mm, 1/125 f5.6, 200 ISO, 3008 x 2000, RAW, tripod

◀ DSLR, 80-200mm lens at 200mm, 1/25 f16, 200 ISO, 3008 x 2000, RAW, tripod

◀ DSLR, 80-200mm lens zoomed, 1/20 f11, 200 ISO, 3008 x 2000, RAW, tripod

FILTERS

There are several filters that can be used to enhance your people pictures, including warming filters for overcast conditions or shade, and cooling filters for early morning or late-evening light. Filters also protect your lenses from dirt, dust, scratches and fingerprints. It's much cheaper to replace a new filter than it is to repair a lens.

Skylight 1A & Ultraviolet (UV) Filters

These filters are most often left on the front of the lens as protective devices. They are useful for slightly cleaning up skin tones by removing the excessive bluishness that often occurs in colour photography outdoors, especially in the open shade. Skylight filters tend to create warmer images because they are usually pinkish, but UV filters are colourless.

80 Series Filters

The 80A, 80B and 80C filters are blue-coloured, colour-conversion filters. They reduce the yellow/orange cast that occurs when using daylight film with incandescent light. If you're going to take a lot of pictures inside using incandescent light (rather than flash) such as stage lighting and don't like the colour cast, the mid-strength 80B is a good option. But be aware it reduces the light reaching the film by one stop.

Entertainers in waiting, Ubud, Bali, Indonesia

In the shadows the skin tones are often cold, so it's a good idea to warm them up. I was lucky enough to be invited to a festival celebrating the blessing of a temple. I saw the performers sitting in the shadows and took a picture of them. In the second image I used an 81B warming filter to ensure a much more acceptable colour.

◀ 35mm SLR, 24mm lens, 1/60 f4, Sensia 200

◀ 35mm SLR, 24mm lens, 1/60 f2.8-f4, Sensia 200, 81B filter

81 Series Filters

The 81A, 81B and 81C filters are amber-coloured, light-balancing filters referred to as warming filters. Essentially strong skylight filters, they're commonly used to reduce the bluish cast from snow scenes and when taking portraits in open shade. The 81C is the strongest of the three and is the one to carry as a good general warming filter. It reduces the light reaching the film by two-thirds of a stop.

82 Series Filters

The 82A, 82B and 82C filters are blue-coloured, light-balancing filters referred to as cooling filters. They reduce the warm tones of early-morning and late-afternoon light to give a more natural look to portraits.

AUTOWINDERS

Most modern compact cameras and SLRs have built-in autowinders that advance the film automatically. If you own an SLR that doesn't have this feature, check your camera manual to see if it's possible to attach an autowinder as an accessory. If you can, it's well worth spending the money as they're particularly useful for photographing people. You can shoot without having to remove your eye from the viewfinder between frames, which lets you keep your eye on the subject and maintain your composition within the frame.

Man wrapped in white, Adjibar, Ethiopia

Sometimes the location dictates the picture. I waited half an hour for a person to appear who looked interesting and was wearing the sort of clothes that fitted with the background. I kept the camera in front of my eye and fired a few frames.

▲ 35mm SLR, 35mm lens, 1/250 f2.8, Sensia 100

TRIPODS

Tripods provide stability for the camera when photographing people in low light; people in action, such as dancers, circus performers or participants in sports and games; people in parades; or when using a long lens. However, they're heavy and inconvenient when you wish to move around. Many people photographers prefer to shoot with faster film rather than be burdened with a tripod.

If you don't want to carry a tripod there are other ways to support your camera. A monopod is a one-legged camera support. It's lighter and less inconvenient than a tripod and can supply the same stability for short exposure times when photographing people, as long as it is held steady and still.

A table-top tripod is a small camera support that you can put on a table or ledge. A cushion, pillow, sleeping bag or bundled coat can also support a camera. A further option is to lean or wedge yourself against a wall or tree, to breathe out gently, and to then fire the shutter: you have made yourself into a very good camera support.

FLASH UNITS

Available light is the primary source of illumination for most of the people photographs you're likely to take on the road, but it still pays to carry a compact flash unit (also called a flashgun or Speedlight). There will be times when it's inconvenient, impractical, prohibited or simply too dark (even for fast films) to set up a tripod. Flash can also be used outdoors to fill in shadows on a person's face.

Fishmonger, Hobart, Australia

The daylight coming through the windows and door of this fishmonger's factory was not quite bright enough for me to shoot a picture. I activated the fill flash mode on my camera and was able to fill in the shadows on the man's face and balance the light in the room.

▲ 35mm SLR, 35mm lens, 1/60 f4, Kodachrome 64 ISO

REFLECTORS

Reflectors reflect or bounce light. They can range from white walls to mirrors, from white towels to newspapers and from bedroom sheets to purpose-made reflector panels of silver, gold or white. They are mainly used to fill in the shadows with light. The reflector is positioned so that the light hits it and bounces back into the shadows on or around your subject.

The advantage of using a reflector instead of a flash is that you can see where the light is changing. By walking around your subject with the reflector you can create different styles of light. Place the reflector on one side of the subject and you will have side lighting. If you place the reflector directly in front of your subject you will acquire a flat and even light.

Dancer, Bali, Indonesia

Balinese dance costumes are beautiful and I always enjoy photographing them. This young dancer posed for me in a room where there was lots of natural light. In the first photograph her skin looks cold and dull. For the second photograph I asked somebody to hold a gold reflector for me. This enhanced the picture and gave the dancer's skin a much brighter look.

▶ 35mm SLR, 85mm lens, 1/60 f5.6-4, Sensia 100

▶▶ 35mm SLR, 85mm lens, 1/60 f4, Sensia 100, gold reflector

FILM

The choice of film is a creative decision which should be made well before you head off to take some serious pictures. Kodak, Fujifilm, Agfa and Ilford make a wide range of film types, some of which are designed specifically for photographing people. Kodak Portra and Fujicolor Superia Reala colour negative films and Fujichrome Astia 100 and Agfachrome RSX II colour transparency films are notable for their accurate skin tones.

Professional photographers tend to endlessly debate the question of what is the best film when really it's a matter of individual taste. Different films record colour and tone differently. Film choice also determines the density of grain (the structure of tiny nodules on the film), which can obscure the detail in the picture. A slow 100 ISO film has less grain and records fine detail. Higher film speeds with more grain don't record the detail as well but can add atmosphere, particularly in low light. A good starting point is to use a 100 ISO film if you want colour slides or a 200 ISO film if you want colour prints from negatives. Try a variety of films under different lighting conditions and see which one gives you the most pleasing results.

The choice will be easier if you know what you want to do with the images you take. If you wish to make prints for an album or to send copies to friends and the people you photograph, then colour negative film is best. If you intend to submit your pictures to a photo library or to license your pictures for publication, then colour transparency film is best.

Women at Prayer, Tehran, Iran

You don't always have to have to look for brightly coloured situations or events to shoot colour photographs. Subdued colour can be equally effective in conveying mood. There is a stillness and peacefulness about these women which is largely conveyed by the muted colours of their clothing.

▲ 35mm SLR, 85mm lens, 1/125 f5.6, Kodachrome 64

A man in costume, Delhi, India
◀ 35mm SLR, 85mm lens, 1/125 f5.6, Ektachrome E100VS

PRINTS OR SLIDES?

The most basic decision to make is whether you want colour prints (negative film), colour slides (transparency film) or black-and-white prints. It's a mistake to think you might satisfactorily carry several cameras loaded with colour negative, black-and-white negative and colour transparency film. To carry even two cameras loaded with different film means you will often be confused and indecisive, sometimes to the point of taking no photographs at all.

Transparency (slide) film can give rich colours and sharp results. Most professional photographers of people use transparencies as they are more suitable for reproduction. But colour negative film is more popular for those who want a record of a trip, images for an album or the ability to make prints easily and cheaply.

Colour negative film is readily available, cheap to purchase and print, and has more flexibility with exposure; that is, you can make mistakes and have them rectified when the film is printed.

Colour Negative Film

Colour negatives can be shot in a greater range of light conditions than transparency film. This is due to the changes which can be made during the printing of the film. If your picture has a colour cast or bias, say blue or green from tungsten or fluorescent light, this bias can be removed. The prints can also be made darker or brighter, warmer or colder (from the cold or blue end of the spectrum to the warm or orange end of the spectrum). Thus colour negative film is the preferred film for compact point-and-shoot cameras. The limitations of the compact camera can be compensated for due to the flexibility of the negative film exposure.

Colour negatives can also be developed and printed in accessible minilabs on your journey. The advantage is that you and others can enjoy your prints of people soon after you take your photographs, and thus have constant feedback on what has been successful. The disadvantage is that you have little or no control over how minilabs develop your negatives and the prints may be inconsistent in colour and tone. The optimal solution is to have all your negatives printed or reprinted at a familiar lab when you return home.

One of the best colour negative films for photographing people is the Fujicolor Superia Reala with a 100 ISO rating; it provides natural skin tones and fine texture.

Colour Transparency Film

Transparency (slide) film gives sharper and clearer images with better colour saturation than negative film. Slides are the closest you can get to the actual photographic experience; that is, the colours and details envisaged by the photographer, rather than something reinterpreted by a technician working on the development and printing of negative film.

Prints can be made from transparency film but the process is more expensive than with colour negatives. To get a high-quality print from a slide, it is always best to take it to a professional lab.

Transparency film comes in a wide variety of stock. It ranges from 100 ISO to 1600 ISO, allowing it to be shot in many different weather and light conditions, indoors as well as outdoors. Some transparency film gives you a high colour saturation, making the reds and

Water festival, Tampaksiring, Bali, Indonesia

There is a wide range of colour slide films available. Each film has its own characteristics and will render the same scene in different colours. One picture was taken with Elitechrome 100; the other was taken with Fujichrome Sensia. Choice of film is a matter of individual personal preference, because everybody sees colour differently.

▲ 35mm SLR, 35mm lens, 1/60 f2.8, Sensia 100

▲ 35mm SLR, 35mm lens, 1/60 f2.8, Elitechrome 100

Monk, Bangkok, Thailand

Not only is the early morning a great time to take pictures but it is the quietest time of day in a major city like Bangkok. Every morning I walked around the pagodas, watching the monks going about their chores. The sun came through the clouds and the light suddenly gave a nice sparkle to this monk's face; it also created interesting shadows on the building behind him. The picture was taken on Kodachrome 64. It is a slow film that has a fine grain and works well in most conditions.

▲ 35mm SLR, 20mm lens, 1/125 f5.6, Kodachrome 64

the blues leap out from the picture. Other types give you a more neutral colour and realistic skin tones. Differences in colour reproduction are greater in slide film than in negative film. Kodak, Agfa and Fujifilm all make a range of colour transparency films and each provides different results. The need to decide which type of film to take on a journey is especially relevant to colour transparency film. Fujichrome Astia 100F, Fujichrome Sensia II, Kodak Ektachrome E100G, Kodak Ektachrome E100SW and Agfachrome RSX II are all transparency films which produce natural skin tones with a neutral colour balance.

Black & White Film

Black-and-white negative film is always an option for photographing people due to its unique ability to capture subtle shades and tones. One of the great advantages of setting up your own darkroom, aside from the complete control you have over the development process, is its cheapness compared to the cost of sending the film off to a professional black-and-white lab (minilabs usually send the film off to the professional labs). A further option is black-and-white chromogenic film, which can be developed by a minilab using the same chemicals and processes as colour negative film, but unfortunately you often get a blue or brown colour cast. A more satisfactory result comes from printing the negative on black-and-white paper.

Kodak T-Max with either the 100 or 400 ISO is a black-and-white film which gives extreme sharpness and fine grain, making it a very good film for people photography.

PUSHING FILM

Pushing film is the technique of setting the ISO on the camera one or two stops higher than the actual ISO rating of the film you are using. It's a useful technique if you are only carrying one type of film and want to take pictures in low light without a tripod or flash. Pushing film causes the camera to underexpose the film. When you take the exposed roll to the lab, you instruct them to process the film at the rating at which you have set it. For example, if you expose a 100 ISO film at 200 ISO, instruct the lab to 'push' the film one stop. Similarly, if you expose a 100 ISO film at 400 ISO, instruct the lab to push the film two stops.

If you do push the film, it will become more grainy and contrasting. But there are films, such as some professional Kodak and Fuji films, that are designed to be pushed with very little change to contrast and grain.

It is recommended to never push any film more than three stops.

Monk blessing girls, Siem Riep, Cambodia

The monk was performing a ritual that involved scooping water and throwing it over these worshippers. I wanted to freeze the action and to capture the atmosphere. I pushed the film two stops to a higher ISO, so I was able to shoot on a faster shutter speed.

◀ 35mm SLR, 85mm lens, 1/250 f2.8, Ektachrome E200 pushed two stops to 800 ISO

PART TWO:

With over six billion people in the world there is no shortage of subject matter for the people photographer. For many travellers, though, the step from seeing someone they would like to photograph to pressing the shutter on a beautifully lit, carefully composed and technically perfect shot doesn't come easily. However, there is a lot you can do before confronting the population of the world with your camera that can help you take the pictures you want. Start with research and practice. Then, at your destination, spend time exploring, as this will provide ideas for locations and subjects. Finally, when you're ready to take some pictures, think about how to approach your subjects; your understanding of photo etiquette will play a considerable part in capturing great pictures.

BEING PREPARED

BEFORE YOU TRAVEL

You will be rewarded with more photo opportunities and better pictures if you take the time to become thoroughly familiar and confident with your equipment and find out as much as you can about your intended destinations before you leave home.

PERFECTING YOUR TECHNIQUE

Your subject's cooperation will be enhanced by your ability to work efficiently.

▸ **It's vitally important to practise photographic techniques that make it easier for you to relate to your subject.**

Hesitating for too long over shutter speeds, apertures, lenses or flashlights is a certain way of ensuring that people become self-conscious. Almost inevitably they will then start adopting a pose. Worse still, they could decide you're wasting their time and turn away.

You should also practise making quick decisions on how best to compose and light your subject. Start by photographing friends and relatives as if you've never seen them before or, conversely, photograph them with all the insights you have into their personality and character. It also helps to photograph them in unfamiliar locations, as this is what you will encounter on the road. Study the results and then take lots more pictures. Learn from each success (how could I have made the image even better?) and improve on every mistake (I won't do that again!).

Woman in traditional Hmong dress, Hobart, Australia

The bright clothes of this young woman from the mountains of Laos are contrasted against the soft hues of her environment. In the first photograph, she is too close to the lens, and the bright colours overwhelm the environment. In the second, I have placed her further away, but the composition is still not correct. In the third, I have asked her to sit and turn so she is in profile. When shooting a portrait on location it's important to ensure the subject and environment are balanced.
Three images 35mm SLR, 24mm lens, 1/125 f8, Kodachrome 64

Woodcarver, Phnom Penh, Cambodia
◀ 35mm SLR, 24mm lens, 1/30 f4, Kodachrome 64 ISO

RESEARCHING YOUR DESTINATION

There are very few places in the world that cannot be researched prior to visiting.

▶ **The more you know about people's backgrounds, the better your chances of taking great photographs when you meet them.**

Travel brochures, film documentaries, fiction and nonfiction literature, pictorial books, guidebooks and the web all provide valuable information. Study the pictures and ask yourself a few questions. What did previous travellers think was worth photographing? What might you do differently? Would you choose a different time of day or different people to photograph? Talk to your friends and friends of friends who have been to the places you plan to go. What were the highlights of their trip? If they took pictures, what photo opportunities did they most enjoy? What did they most regret missing?

It's best you don't miss such opportunities yourself. Research the dates of festivals, fiestas, carnivals, bullfights, parades, shows and public events held in the countries you're visiting. Few things are worse than getting there a day or two after the event. Imagine hearing other travellers and local people discussing fantastic dancers at a carnival or gravity-defying gymnasts at an international circus that has now departed. 'You should have been there' are the last words a travelling photographer ever wants to hear.

Aside from special events, there are other things to research. Do the people of your host country possess unique occupations, arts or crafts? Are there unusual national icons, sites of religion or monuments that could be used as backgrounds for portraits? What will the weather be like? Are the days likely to be sunlit or overcast? These factors will help you decide what sort of film you'll need and what kind of lenses or other accessories you should take. Research will also help you decide how long to stay and what to do with your time.

Good research can also reward you on a more subtle basis. Is it a culture of easy-going and relaxed informality, of rushed 'busyness' or of strict formality and punctuality? How might this culture be reflected by your choice of subjects and the locations in which you depict people?

On a more mundane level, knowing about attitudes to time can save you much frustration. In some cultures, typically in the West, time is measured by clocks and watches, and is regarded as the way to arrange appointments.

Salt seller, Shiraz, Iran

I saw this salt vendor by the side of the road in Iran. We established a rapport after I sat down and talked to him, through my interpreter, about his life as a farmer. All over the world I have found that if you take the time to talk to people in the countryside they are usually friendly, warm and very happy to pose for a photograph.

▶ 35mm SLR, 24mm lens, 1/125 f5.6, Kodachrome 64

But in other cultures time can be regarded with equal legitimacy as a sort of seamless flow in which things happen when the mood feels right. In these cultures, be prepared to wait when you turn up on time for an advertised event. An elephant riders' parade in Asia may be supposed to start at dawn but might actually commence late in the afternoon. A twilight drumming competition in Africa may begin not at dusk but late at night, when the drummers are ready.

Through your research you may find out that in some countries it is culturally impolite to refuse a request, especially if it comes from a guest in one's home and/or country. Sometimes people may agree to a photo session but will fail to keep the appointment. Researching the culture beforehand will help you understand why this can happen and also possibly alert you to other nonverbal gestures which indicate that 'yes' actually means 'no'.

Culture is embodied in language. Simply learning a few local words and phrases will make you welcome anywhere, and learning the nonverbal signs will show that you understand local customs. In some countries, you should never sit with your feet pointing at the person you are speaking with. In other countries you must take off your shoes before going into a mosque or a temple; yet in another country this may be considered ostentatious or foolish. These differences will provide endless inspiration and subject matter for your photography.

AT YOUR DESTINATION

When you arrive in a new place, get out and have a look around, camera in hand. The quicker you get your bearings and meet some of the locals the better.

EXPLORING YOUR SURROUNDINGS

The most rewarding activity upon arrival is to go out for a walk, carrying a camera with your favourite lens.

▸ **Fresh eyes see extraordinary things which after just a few days can start to seem ordinary.**

Go to the locations you've researched and confirm what you learned about them. Check out the light there. Would it be better in the morning or afternoon? What would be the best angle from which to shoot? Get a feel for the people and their activities. When do people congregate? What sort of people are they? What sorts of activities happen here?

Always have your camera ready and don't hesitate to use it. During these first few days it's highly likely you'll photograph a number of people who seem new or exotic. Don't fight the temptation. The people *are* new and exotic, and your fresh eyes are providing deep insights. Quite often your best picture will be one of those taken during the first days in a new place.

Street Barber, Hanoi, Vietnam

As soon as I check into my hotel I unpack a camera and walk around the streets to get a feel for the place. A hundred yards away from my hotel I found this local barber setting up his stool and mirror under the shade of a tree. I returned later in the day when the light was better and the barber had a customer who didn't mind being photographed having a quick trim and shave.

◀ DSLR, 35-70mm lens at 52mm, 1/60 F4.5, 200 ISO, 3008 x 2000, RAW

Portrait of young girl, Melaka, Malaysia
◀ DSLR, 35-70mm lens at 52mm, 1/200 F3.5, 200 ISO, 3008 x 2000, RAW

APPROACHING PEOPLE

Travellers are often daunted by the apparent obstacles between seeing a potential photograph and capturing it on film or memory card. Where possible, try and create space in your trip where you can spend time relating to your subjects. This allows you to understand the context in which they live and encourages them to relax in your presence. However, time constraints when travelling don't always allow for this approach and you'll often want to photograph people with whom you haven't had the opportunity to connect, so confidence in approaching people and communicating what you want to do becomes very important.

Good interpersonal skills – the ability to communicate effectively and warmly, both verbally and nonverbally – are essential for successful people photography. Not everybody can walk up to total strangers, ask permission to photograph them and then within minutes have them ceasing work, shifting position or adjusting their clothing. But possessing a good understanding of cultural differences and knowing how much can be conveyed through sign language, mime and humour will get you a long way.

Photo Etiquette

In some areas of the world people are convinced that a camera can steal their soul or spirit. In other places there are deep concerns about how and where pictures of people may be used. For example, a large number of Aboriginal people in Australia are bound by strong laws against seeing an image of any dead relative. There are also dances and rituals in Aboriginal societies that are secret 'men's business' or 'women's business' – outsiders, as

Indian women, Samode, India

The lady in the picture opposite agreed to be photographed only if all the female members of her family were photographed together in a group. The other part of the agreement was that I would send her a copy of the picture.

▲ 35mm SLR, 85mm lens, 1/125 f5.6, Sensia 100

▶ 35mm SLR, 35mm lens, 1/125 f8, Sensia 100

well as the female or male tribespeople (depending on whose business it is), are forbidden to witness these activities.

▶ **Capturing the most memorable image is not justified if it means transgressing cultural or religious beliefs.**

Principled photographers bear these sorts of things in mind. There are photographs in existence which should never have been taken. Religious and spiritual privacy should be sacrosanct. So should the rights of children and other people whose images could be exploited even if the photographer never intended any exploitation to occur. There is no written code of ethics as a guide to individual behaviour; instead, it is a matter of one's own value system.

It is usually considered ethical, and is nearly always practical, to ask permission before taking someone's picture. There are circumstances, such as in candid photography, crowds, street scenes or at festivals, when seeking permission is unnecessary. But not asking permission from an individual or a small group can cause deep offence. It may also result in considerable difficulties for other photographers. In practical terms, it will severely limit what you might otherwise achieve. People can turn away from you or glare at the camera with obvious resentment. A photograph of people who clearly do not wish to have their picture taken is not an image you will be proud to take home.

Gaining Permission

The reality is that many photographs require direct interaction between the photographer and the subject, which usually begins with asking someone if they mind having their photograph taken. Many travellers are self-conscious about seeking the cooperation of people they've never met and will never see again. They may dread being misunderstood or having their intentions misinterpreted. They may feel guilty if the people they wish to photograph are poverty-stricken. None of this does travellers any discredit. In fact, their own sensitivity can sometimes make them move on, even when people are perfectly willing and pleased to be photographed.

But there is no harm in asking. Language is not a barrier in seeking permission. Eye contact, and a smile whilst holding up a camera, is almost always enough. A refusal, if firm or vehement, should be accepted with grace. But a slight shake of the head with a smile matching your own smile may signify something else. There could be cultural or religious reasons why this is neither the time nor the place for a photograph. In any case, stay polite and non-aggressive. Photographer James Marshall has rightly said, 'As photographers, we deal in a universal language. Use your knowledge of this to your advantage while on location. Your body language, comfort level, warmth and positive attitude in dealing with potential photo subjects anywhere in the world will make all the difference as to whether you do come home with that absolute winning image. Treat people with respect, openness and honesty wherever you go. And try to give something back, even if it's just a sincere handshake and a big-hearted smile.'

Posing & Composing

Always approach your subject with confidence, as this will inspire their confidence and increase cooperation. Often this will be enhanced if you explain what you're doing as you

Woman peeking at camera, Abhaneri, India

This veiled Indian woman agreed to be photographed but then lifted a corner of her veil to watch what was happening. The photograph captures the moment when she did so. She was well aware that I was photographing her face, and had a delightful fit of giggles when I ceased taking pictures.

▲ 35mm SLR, 85mm lens, 1/250 f5.6, Sensia 100

do it. This comes across as a greatly appreciated effort to relate and communicate with the person or people you're photographing, who, like you, desire a memorable image.

▶ **It's amazing what can be achieved through courtesy, friendliness and good humour.**

You will capture better, more spontaneous images if you make some creative and technical decisions before approaching your subject. Consider what you are trying to say about the person or people, the visual story you are trying to tell and why you are taking the photograph. For example, if you wished to photograph a camel trader at the Pushkar Camel Fair in Rajasthan, India, then you would probably be wanting to tell a story of colour, vibrancy and energy. So you would look for a trader who is personable, happy and physically exuberant.

Think about how you want to photograph your subject before gaining permission. Should the composition be vertical or horizontal, close-up? A three-quarter view or full-length shot? Would it be best in colour or in black and white? Answering these questions in advance will reduce the amount of time you're asking the subject to contribute to the photographic process. Next, observe how the light is falling on the subject's face and decide where you will take the photo from. This may mean you need to move your subject to a position where the light or background is more suitable. You may want them to change their stance or adjust an item of clothing. Something as simple as getting a person to remove a piece of white cotton from a black coat can mean the difference between a mediocre picture and a good one. So can asking a companion, partner or child to move to the side. If you do need to move someone or something it's often not a good idea to physically touch people, unless you have established a good rapport (and it's usually always a bad idea if they are of the opposite sex). Instead, you might demonstrate a pose you wish them to take, perhaps the position in which you first saw them, by imitating the pose yourself. If your subject is wearing a hat that is covering their eyes try miming to show that you want it moved or removed.

When you're ready to take the photo, be aware of what the subject is doing. Are they continuing the activity which first attracted your attention? Are they following you with their eyes when you want them to look elsewhere? Have they blinked at the very instant you clicked the camera? When in doubt, take a second, third or fourth frame. People tend to pose for the first photograph and then relax into a more natural position after the first click of the shutter. They might blink, close their eyes, look away or change expression on your first shot. It's best if you don't pause or take the camera from your eye, so you can capture a quick succession of moments. Autowinders on film cameras are very useful because you don't have to take the camera from your eye to wind the film on.

Paying For Photos

The most common ethical dilemma for travellers is whether or not to pay people for being photographed. It's an area where virtually every piece of advice has to be qualified. Probably the simplest rule is to not offer money unless asked. But if you're asked, the temptation to say 'yes' can be as strong as the urge to say 'no'. The 'yes' might derive from a wish to take the picture as quickly as possible or from sympathy with the poverty of the person whom you wish to photograph. The 'no' might come from the realisation that by paying

Masai man, Nairobi, Kenya

This man asked for a single American dollar before being photographed. I thought it was a fair price to pay for his time and patience. The picture was shot from low down with a wide-angle lens. His stick and robe help to balance the image in the shape of a triangle.

▲ 35mm SLR, 20mm lens, 1/125 f5.6, Kodachrome 64

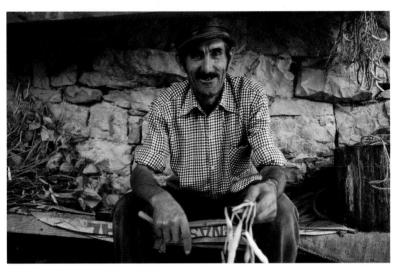

Farmer, Fatima, Portugal

This farmer was initially wary about being photographed but I smiled at him, gestured to my camera and mimed the action of taking of a photograph. He nodded and smiled back. His smile then never left his weather-beaten face.

▲ 35mm SLR, 24mm lens, 1/60 f4, Kodachrome 64

you're making things difficult for the travellers who follow as they will inevitably meet with demands for a similar payment, which soon becomes an expected fee.

The question of payment usually boils down to a matter of judgment on a case-by-case basis. You may feel it's appropriate to pay farmers, tradespeople and street entertainers who have given up time that could have been spent earning a living. A donation to a church or temple might also be merited if you have entered and used it for an environmental portrait.

On the other hand some people who have willingly donated their time can see an offer of money as an insult. They've enjoyed the experience as much as you have and don't want it reduced to a commercial transaction. What they may appreciate, however, is a print of the image. Never forget that many people in the developing world don't have pictures of themselves or their loved ones. If you promise to send them a photograph, make sure you honour the promise. The relationship between the photographer and the subject in such a case is one of genuine mutual benefit.

In the final analysis, you always have a choice. How strongly do you really wish to photograph a particular person? If confronted by a request for payment, you're free to gracefully decline and travel on to photograph someone else.

Model Releases

A model release is a statement signed by the subject of a photograph (or signed by their parent/guardian). It grants permission to the photographer to use the photograph in any way unless it is illegal or defamatory. The subject understands the photograph may be changed or altered but waives the right to inspect the final copy and to lodge a claim for financial remuneration.

Generally, without model releases, images can be licensed for editorial use to magazines, newspapers and books but should not be used for advertising or promotional purposes. Much larger returns are possible for pictures used in advertising, so a signed model release can be very valuable.

Photographers usually ask people to sign model releases when they believe a particular photograph has definite advertising or promotional potential, such as an image of someone appealing or attractive. If you have spent considerable time befriending a subject, gaining trust and cooperation, it can be uncomfortable to then produce a legal document. You can cause suspicion and hurt as people start to wonder how much money you are going to make from the sale of their image. Carry model releases but use them sparingly and sensitively.

These sample releases can be copied onto your own letterhead and adapted for your use. As every situation is different you may want to get some more information and advice about what you need for your particular subject and use. For example, if you're going to use images for non-editorial purposes, bear in mind you may need to provide some compensation (even nominal) for the release to be enforceable – the second sample form provides for this.

MODEL RELEASE

By signing this document:

I irrevocably consent to the Photographer (and its licensees and assigns) incorporating my image or likeness in photographs or illustrations in any form or media (images) and reproducing, publishing and communicating the Images in any form and media for any purpose, whether commercial or otherwise (including advertising), and to the use of my name and any other text or works in connection with the Images. I waive any right to inspect or approve the Images or any publication incorporating the Images and any right to compensation for the use of the Images by the Photographer, its licensees and assigns. I release the Photographer, its licensees and assigns from any or all claims, actions, proceedings, demands and expenses and other liability that may arise in connection with the use of the Images by any person. I confirm that I am either over 18 years of age or that my parent or guardian has also agreed to these terms by signing in the space provided below.

I understand and agree to the above.

Signed: _____   Signed by parent/guardian: _____

Print name: _____   Print name: _____

Address/email/phone number: _____

_____   Date: _____

Description of image: _____

_____

MODEL RELEASE

Photographer: Name: _____

                  Address: _____

In return for valuable consideration received, namely _____ [describe]:

I irrevocably consent to the Photographer (and its licensees and assigns) incorporating my image or likeness in photographs or illustrations in any form or media (images) and reproducing, publishing and communicating the Images in any form and media for any purpose, whether commercial or otherwise (including advertising), and to the use of my name and any other text or works in connection with the Images. I waive any right to inspect or approve the Images or any publication incorporating the Images and any right to compensation for the use of the Images by the Photographer, its licensees and assigns. I release the Photographer, its licensees and assigns from any or all claims, actions, proceedings, demands and expenses and other liability that may arise in connection with the use of the Images by any person. I confirm that I am either over 18 years of age or that my parent or guardian has also agreed to these terms by signing in the space provided below.

I understand and agree to the above.

Signed: _____   Signed by parent/guardian: _____

Print Name: _____   Print name: _____

Address: _____

Date: _____

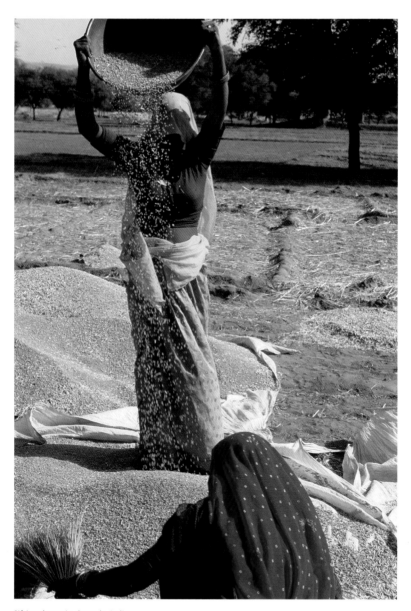

Sifting the grain, Samode, India

The colourful saris of these women were irresistible. But standing still for photographs took up time which they could have spent actively working. I paid a small amount of money, which they were quite happy to accept as compensation.

▲ 35mm SLR, 35mm lens, 1/125 f8, Ektachrome E100G

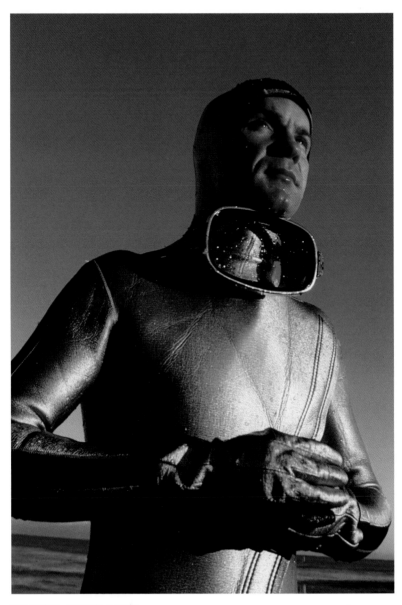

Diver at dawn, Fremantle, Australia

Scouting for a location, preparation and a cooperative subject helped me get the image of this silver-suited diver at sunrise. This is the type of image that could be used many times over so I made sure that I acquired a model release from the subject.

▲ 35mm SLR, 20mm lens, 1/125 f8, Kodachrome 64

PART THREE:

A popular truism among photographers states that cameras don't take pictures, people do. Modern cameras make many things easy but an understanding of the technical elements of photography will mean you can control the exposure, shutter speed, aperture and depth of field to create images that accurately reflect the scene that attracted you to press the shutter in the first place. Once you're confident with your equipment you can concentrate on composition and light, the other key elements that contribute to creating great pictures.

TECHNICAL
ELEMENTS

Aboriginal youth, Daintree Rainforest, Australia
◀ 35mm SLR, 35-70mm lens at 70mm, 1/15 f4, Sensia 100, tripod

EXPOSURE

Exposing your film or sensor to just the right amount of light to create an image with the density of colour you require is the aim every time you press the shutter. There is no universal right or wrong exposure. Like so much in photography, it's a matter of individual choice. Yet pictures can be clearly too dark (underexposed) or too light (overexposed). A good starting point when photographing people is to take the exposure reading from the subject's face. If possible, use a spot meter or utilise a zoom lens to get in very close for a more accurate reading. This will eliminate the possibility of other elements in the scene (such as clothing or background) influencing the light meter.

Flautist, Hobart, Australia

I had been to this location on the previous evening to check when the sun would be in the right position, as I wanted the light of the fading sun to reflect on the face of the flautist. If I had pointed the light meter towards the sun I would have received a false light reading. The solution was to take a spot reading from the subject's face and to bracket the exposures.

◀ 35mm SLR, 35mm lens, Kodachrome 64

Chinatown at night, Singapore

My assignment was to capture the atmosphere of Chinatown in Singapore and to also create a sense of location. I found a place that looked down on the market and set up a table-top tripod on a wall. I waited until around sunset when the exposure of the skyline was balanced with the exposure of the marketplace. At this time of day you have to work fast because the sun drops very quickly and the light and the exposure change just as rapidly.

▲ 35mm SLR, 20mm lens, 1/4 f2.8, Ektachrome E100SW, table-top tripod

Young Woman, Majete, Ethiopia
◀ 35mm SLR, 85mm lens, 1/60 f4, Ektachrome E100VS

Accurate exposure is achieved through the interrelationship between the ISO of the film or sensor setting, shutter speed and aperture. The ideal minimum shutter speed for capturing sharp, hand-held photographs of people is around 1/125 of a second. With slower shutter speeds you run the risk of subject movement and unintentional blur of your subject. A good standard aperture is f8. It will render all the features of an individual sharp and it provides enough depth of field to also record most groups in focus. However, a more considered approach to the combination of shutter speed and aperture, on an image-by-image basis, will let you create more interesting and varied images and access the creative possibilities of intentional blur and controlling depth of field (see Composition, p67).

If you have the chance to take more than one frame of your subject, it's often worth bracketing your exposures half a stop either side of the camera's recommended meter reading to ensure you get the exposure you're after. It's particularly useful when the light is contrasting and you're using colour transparency film, which has very little exposure latitude. If there is significant contrast between the subject's clothes and background, shoot several extra frames at a full stop over and a full stop under, just to be certain of capturing your image.

Men at sports club, Tehran, Iran

These men are warming up for a game of *warzesh bastani*. For both images, I used a tripod as I wanted to capture the details of the sporting centre. In the first picture, I waited until the players were still and used an exposure of 1/15 of a second, so the players are sharp. In the second image the men are blurred because they were moving and I used an exposure of 1/4 of a second.

◀ 35mm SLR, 24mm lens, 1/15 f2.8, Kodachrome 64, tripod

◀ 35mm SLR, 24mm lens, 1/4 f4, Kodachrome 64, tripod

Cooking satay, Singapore

It was important to capture the fanning of the fire. I put the camera on a tripod, used a slow shutter speed and underexposed the flash by one stop; that way the flash wasn't the dominating light.

◀ 35mm SLR, 24mm lens, 1/8 f8, Fijicolour NPH 400, tripod

Baptism in Jordan River, Yardenit, Israel

The light meter was confused by the contrast between the dark blue river and the whiter gowns of the people being baptised. Bracketing revealed that the correct exposure was half a stop less than what the meter was reading.

◀ 35mm SLR, 35-70mm lens at 70mm, 1/125 f4, Sensia 100

▲ 35mm SLR, 35mm lens, 1/15 f4, Ektachrome E100GX, tripod and reflector, I/2 stop overexposed

▲ 35mm SLR, 35mm lens, 1/15 f4-5.6, Ektachrome E100GX, tripod and reflector, correct exposure

▲ 35mm SLR, 35mm lens, 1/15 f5.6, Ektachrome E100GX, tripod and reflector, I/2 stop underexposed

Dancer, Siem Riep, Cambodia

A lot of photographers like to expose their images slightly darker than the meter suggests and bracketing is a good way of achieving this. Usually out of three bracketed exposures there is one I like and one that is perfectly acceptable. In these three images, taken with the use of a light meter, the first is half a stop overexposed, the second one is correctly exposed and the third is half a stop underexposed.

COMPOSITION

Composition is the way in which all the elements within an image relate to each other. Good composition results in an image that presents your subject in exactly the way you envisaged. Think about the person you're going to photograph and ask yourself why you're taking their picture and what you're trying to show. If in doubt, keep your compositions simple by filling the frame with your subject or by excluding excessive clutter that will distract the viewer from focussing on your subject. Composition is an art that can be studied in books of photographs and paintings, and by spending time in galleries and museums. The key variables to consider as you compose a photograph are subject placement, depth of field, framing, viewpoint, content selection, orientation, focus and choice of lens.

Hindu ceremony, Singapore

The frame is filled, from the man's face on the left to the man's face on the right. When you fill the frame, the challenge is to make sure you only include the amount of detail you require. Remember to scan the edges of the frame for unnecessary objects when you're looking through your viewfinder.

◀ DSLR, 17-35mm lens at 17mm, 1/60 f9, 200 ISO, 2240 x 1488, JPEG

Gauchos, Hucal, Argentina

I was camping on the Pampas with a group of gauchos. After work finished at the end of the day they would eat, drink and play music. The accordion in the hands of the gaucho is the centre of the picture. By only including a portion of the other musicians your eye is led immediately to the main point of interest in the image.

▲ 35mm SLR, 24mm lens, 1/60 f4, Sensia 100

Tao priest, Singapore

◀ 35mm SLR, 85mm lens, 1/125 f4, Ektachrome E200

SUBJECT PLACEMENT

The great artists of the past discovered that by placing the main elements of a composition at points one-third of the way from the edges of the frame their paintings became more dynamic and interesting. This technique is known as the 'rule of thirds' and is a very practical place to start when deciding how to compose a photograph. It helps prevent the great temptation of going for the 'bull's-eye'; that is, placing your subject in the dead centre of the picture. Resulting images are often boring and static, as the eye is drawn to the centre of the frame and stays there, taking in little else in the picture. When filling the frame with a close-up of a person's face, try placing their eyes one-third from the top of the frame. When taking environmental portraits, place the subject's head away from the centre of the frame and your pictures will instantly look a lot less static.

The auto-focus systems on many cameras are constructed with the focus and exposure sensors in the middle of the viewfinder, and this is often the reason subjects are placed in the centre of the frame. Most cameras, including compacts, have a focus-lock facility that you should become comfortable in using so the technology doesn't impede your ability to compose creatively.

Statue and priest at Hindu temple, Singapore

In the first photograph, the subject's head is in the centre of the frame or the bull's-eye. The diagonal lines of the roof beams lead the eye away from him. The chair and scraps of rubbish are further distractions. I took the second photograph after removing the junk and standing on a chair to shoot from a different angle. The priest's head is now in the bottom third of the image. The blank spaces of the first photograph have gone and the statue is more relevant.

▲ DSLR, 17-35mm lens at 17mm, 1/250 f5.6, 200 ISO, 3008 x 2000, RAW

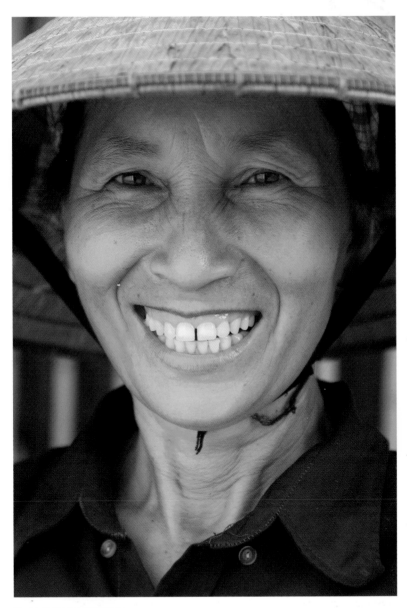

Street vendor, Hanoi, Vietnam

It is just as important to use the rule of thirds when photographing portraits. When you look at this picture your gaze should go immediately to the subject's eyes which are placed in the top one third of the picture. I indicated to this woman in sign language to lift up her hat a little so that her face was not covered in shadow.

▲ DSLR, 35-70mm lens at 52mm, 1/250 F3.5, 200 ISO, 3008 x 2000, RAW

DEPTH OF FIELD

Depth of field is the area of a photograph that is in focus and acceptably sharp. It's one of the most valuable creative tools at the photographer's disposal and plays an integral part in creating images that reflect the photographer's intent. Depth of field is determined by the aperture setting. A wide aperture of f2 or f4 will throw the background of your portraits out of focus and isolate your subject from the environment, often with very pleasing results. If you stop down to a smaller aperture such as f11 or f16 you will record the subject and their environment in sharp focus. When shooting environmental portraits, or groups of people, aim for an aperture of at least f8 to ensure that everyone is in focus.

Indian soldiers in red, Delhi, India

These soldiers were relaxing before they marched at the Indian Independence Day celebration. When using a wide-angle lens you should try to get everything in focus. I photographed these soldiers with a wide-angle lens and a reasonably slow shutter speed which provided the large aperture required. The resulting image is sharp from edge to edge.

▲ 35mm SLR, 20mm lens, 1/60 f11, Kodachrome 64

**Boatmen,
Hotaquai, Guyana**

Never let bad weather
stop you from taking
pictures. I closed the lens
down to an aperture of
f16 so the focus would
extend from the man
in the front of the boat
to the man in the back.
If you want to achieve
great depth of field, make
sure you stop the lens
down as far as you can.

◀ 35mm SLR, 20mm lens,
1/60 f16, TRI-X 400

Composition Depth of Field   71

FRAMING

The use of foreground material to frame a person offers interesting creative possibilities. Well-executed framing brings a three-dimensional feel to a photograph as it leads the viewer's eye towards the subject. Doorways, archways, windows and tree branches are commonly used as frames. Be careful not to select a frame that is more dominant or interesting than the subject. Framing also becomes less interesting if it's used in a whole series of images, so make sure you vary your compositions.

Bridesmaid with umbrella, Siem Riep, Cambodia

The face of the bridesmaid is framed between the spokes of her umbrella as she glances back over her shoulder. Don't always look for the obvious; try to find a different angle.

◀ 35mm SLR, 35mm lens, 1/125 f4, Sensia 100

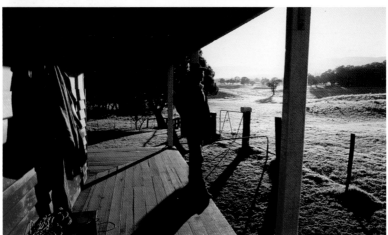

Stockman, Mansfield, Australia

The stockman is framed by the wall, roof and porch beam of his farmhouse. His shadow is the pivot of the image, leading the eye to his figure as he stands in profile with a rim of light around the upper part of his body.

▲ 35mm SLR, 24mm lens, 1/250 f4, Sensia 100

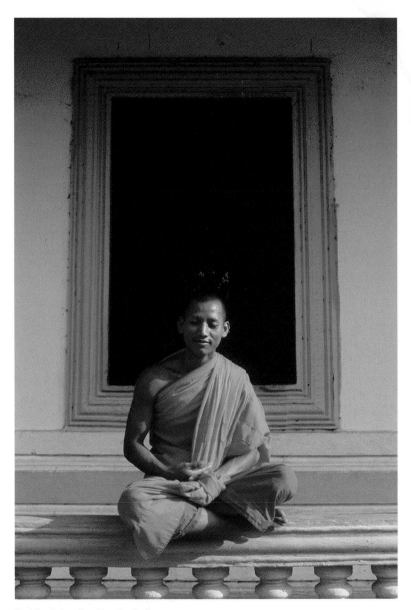

Monk in window, Siem Riep, Cambodia

The first frame is provided by the floor posts. The second frame is the window. There is another smaller window behind the monk's head. The light from this small window ensures that his head doesn't disappear into the black background. A frame within a frame gives a sense of meditation, a world within a world.

▲ 35mm SLR, 24mm lens, 1/250 f5.6, Ektachrome E100G.

VIEWPOINT

Varying your viewpoint is an easy way to improve compositions. Holding the camera to your eye when in a standing position is only one of many options. Try crouching down,

lying on the ground, going down on one knee or standing up on something for a higher point of view. Try moving slightly to the left or right; even one step in any direction can make a big difference and you may find a more interesting viewpoint. Many inexperienced photographers make the mistake of stepping back when they should move forwards. The great photo-journalist Robert Capa made the point when he said, 'If your pictures are not good enough, it means you're not close enough.'

Chinese temple, Singapore

The first photograph really shows nothing but brown tiles. So I changed my position and found an opportunity to take a more interesting photograph. Outside the temple there were red and yellow flowers on a flower cart that matched the red and gold of the temple and I used these as a frame. Changing your viewpoint can help you create a very different vision of a place.

◀ DSLR, 17-35mm lens at 19mm, 1/125 f6.3, 400 ISO,
▼ 3008 x 2000, RAW

Man with iguana, Melaka, Malaysia

The main square of Melaka is nearly always busy with tourists, market stalls and brightly coloured rickshaws. The town has a mixture of local and European architecture, and the market place is a great backdrop. Remember to fill your frame with only what you want to show; if you include too much your subject will be lost in the background.

This wide image shows the man with an iguana but includes too much background, and the people wandering around are a distraction.

◀ DSLR, 35-70mm lens at 35mm, 1/200 f6.3, 200 ISO, 3008 x 2000, RAW

By changing the viewpoint, moving slightly to the left and zooming in for a close-up image, all of the unnecessary background is cut out and clearly identifies the man being photographed with the iguana as the subject matter.

▲ DSLR, 35-70mm lens at 62mm, 1/200 f7.1, 200 ISO, 3008 x 2000, RAW

CONTENT SELECTION

Every element and detail that you include in your composition should lead the viewer's eye to the subject's face and eyes. Straight, curved, parallel or vertical lines such as roof lines, light poles, walls and clothing can be used to achieve this compositional goal. If they don't work in this way you have two options: move the subject to another position or change your viewpoint.

Always scan the entire frame before you press the shutter release to make sure there are no distracting elements behind the subject, such as light poles apparently growing out of the subject's head, or the edge of a table protruding into the corner of the frame. Use the camera's depth-of-field preview button (if it has one) to double-check, as it will bring into sharp focus unwanted elements.

Tao monks, Singapore

I was so impressed with the colour of the robes worn by these female Tao monks that I came back three times. It's a good idea to shoot from different angles – front, side, back – to capture the atmosphere of the ritual.

Two images 35mm SLR, 85mm lens, 1/125 f4, Ektachrome E200

Laughing girls, Melaka, Malaysia

These girls were eager for me to take their photograph. They were such a contrast to the lovely old buildings in Melaka's Chinatown that I couldn't resist taking their picture. For the first shot the girls automatically went into a pose which made a pretty but uninteresting picture. Suddenly they all fell about laughing and I captured a much more spontaneous and lively photograph.

▲ DSLR, 17-35mm lens at 35mm, 1/250 f8, 200 ISO, 3008 x 2000, RAW

Woman with prayer sticks, Hong Kong, China

As this woman prayed I moved in close to fill the frame with her hands and the prayer sticks.

▲ DSLR, 35-70mm lens at 70mm, 1/125 f5, 200 ISO, 3008 x 2000, RAW

ORIENTATION

Though it is much easier to hold the camera horizontally, you should always consider vertical (portrait) framing. It's especially useful when photographing an individual, as it's easier to fill the frame with your subject, whether you are shooting a close-up or full-length picture.

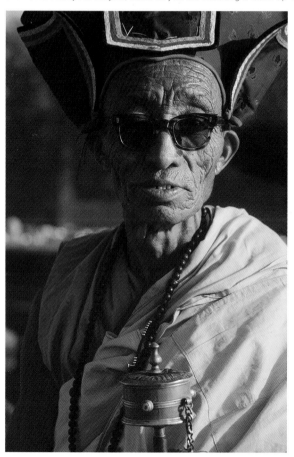

Buddhist Monk, Delhi, India.

This monk was standing was standing in the middle of a crowd of people. By turning the camera to a vertical position, using a medium sized telephoto lens and getting in tight so I could fill the frame, it was possible to isolate him and make a simple but colourful image.

▲ 35mm, 85mm lens, 1/125, f5.6, Ektachrome E100VS

Water hole, Balgo, Australia

This water hole is popular and there is always someone there in the afternoon. So I sat on the riverbank and waited for a photo opportunity.

▶ 35mm SLR, 85mm lens, 1/500 f8, TRI-X 400

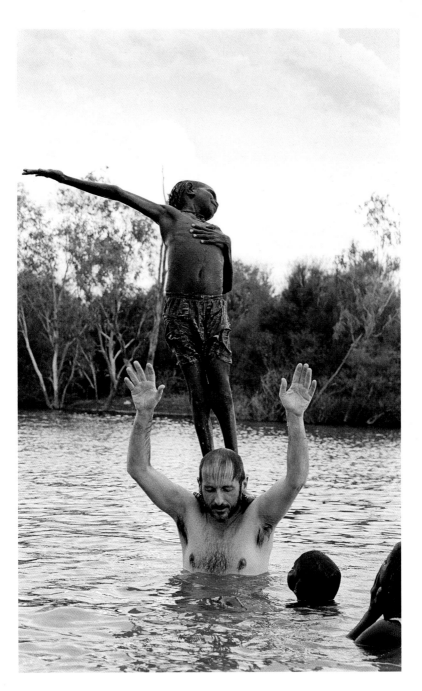

FOCUS

What you focus on will determine where the viewer's eye will rest so it's important to focus accurately. With people photography the simple rule is to focus on your subject's eyes. Even if everything else is out of focus, including their nose and ears, you'll still have a successful picture. Occasionally, a deliberately out-of-focus subject might seem desirable, but usually the photograph will lose impact if the intended subject is out of focus.

Woman praying with monks, Melaka, Malaysia.

The Cheng Hoon Teng Temple is a beautiful temple and the only sound to be heard in the early morning was the chant of the monks. I stood behind this woman who was praying, framed her in the corner of my viewfinder and focused on the praying monks. Because she is out of focus, the woman fills up a space but also forces your eyes across to the main focal point in the picture, the chanting monks.

▲ DSLR, 17-35mm lens at 28mm, 1/30 f2.8, 640 ISO, 3008 x 2000, RAW

Two mullahs, Qom, Iran

After walking around a pool at a mosque in Qom, Iran's centre of Islamic learning, I worked out the best place for a picture. I focussed on a spot at the edge of the pool and waited until these men walked into the frame.

▶ 35mm SLR, 85mm lens, 1/250 f5.6, Kodachrome 64

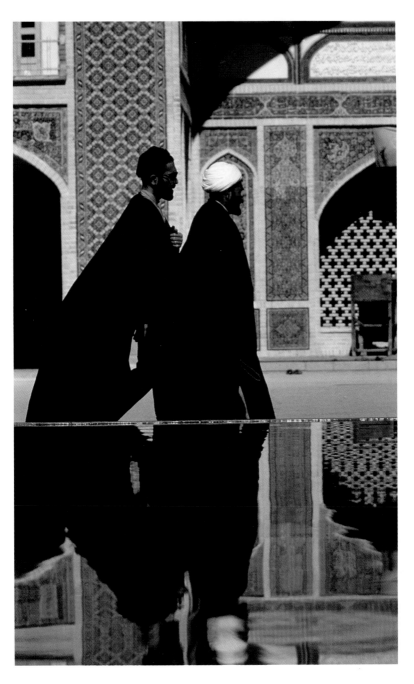

CHOICE OF LENS

As already discussed, you can photograph people with any lens, but your choice will have an impact on your composition. Lenses determine angle or field of view, subject size, depth of field and perspective. A wide-angle lens is great for getting everybody into the picture but if you're not close enough to your subjects they can appear to be an insignificant part of the image. If you get too close, people near the edges of the frame may be unnaturally distorted. However, wide-angle lenses have a greater inherent depth of field than telephoto lenses. Telephoto lenses allow you to shoot at a greater distance from your subject but this may result in a foreshortening or telescopic effect, in which people in the background seem too close to the people in the foreground. See p29 for more information on the features of different types of lenses.

Woman in car, New Zealand

There is no right or wrong lens. Select the lens that helps you create the picture you want to take. The first picture, showing most of the car, was taken with a 20mm lens. The second, which is a much tighter shot of the woman, was taken with a 35mm lens. Lens choice depends on what you think is important and what you want to say.

▲ 35mm SLR, 20mm lens, 1/125
 f4, Ektachrome E100SW

▶ 35mm SLR, 35mm lens, 1/125
 f4, Ektachrome E100SW

LIGHT

The word 'photography' means light drawing. Light etches the image onto film or the pixels of a sensor. Working with light, and not against it, is the essence of good photographic practice. The wise photographer befriends light, understands it and respects it: befriends it because it can be one's greatest assistant; understands it because of its ever-changing qualities; respects it because it is the major element with which to work.

Most of the people pictures you take will be with daylight, but you also need to be confident when photographing with flash and incandescent light. No matter what the light source, look for the key components of colour, quality and direction.

Colour, shape, form, tones and many other essential components depend on the colour, direction and quality of light. Becoming a good photographer of people means you also become a shadow chaser (or light chaser). Shadows allow you to sculpt form around your subjects, and to lead the viewer's eye to your chosen point of interest.

Chinese musicians, Singapore

Learning to work with light is one of the secrets of good photography. I was lucky enough to be able to stand next to these musicians and photograph them performing during a show in a Chinese theatre. To make this picture work I had to wait until the stage lighting on the musicians' faces was balanced with the light on their music sheets. I also needed to be patient enough to wait until there was sufficient light on the audience. To make sure that the colour was correct I switched the lighting mode on my digital camera to tungsten light.

▲ DSLR, 17-35mm lens at 17mm, 1/30 f2.8, 800 ISO, 3008 x 2000, RAW

Spot-lighting wildlife in the Daintree Rainforest, Queensland, Australia

It was raining as we drove through the rainforest at night looking for nocturnal creatures. I asked the guide and one of the tourists to stand in the front of the car we were travelling in and point their torches up into the trees at the birds. The mist and the rain lit by the torches and headlights created a soft and eerie light. Even if it is raining and at night by being resourceful with lighting it is still possible to create interesting pictures of people.

◄ 35mm SLR 35-70mm lens at 70mm, 1/4 f5.6, Fuji Sensia 100, tripod

NATURAL LIGHT

Colour

The sun is the source of all natural light and its colours run up and down the colour spectrum during the day. The sun is low in the sky in the one or two hours after sunrise and before sunset. The sunlight at that stage is at the warm end of the colour spectrum due to the length of the sun's rays. This is a good time for photographing people, as the light's orange hue gives a richer colour to the subject's face. But as the sun reaches the middle of the day the light becomes cooler, creating a blue tinge.

If you don't like the rich warm colours created by the low sun it is possible to cool the light with one of the 80 series filters. The 80A, 80B and 80C are blue-coloured conversion filters and are used for removing the orange/red cast.

Quality

Light quality and mood, characterised by terms such as soft light, harsh light and contrasting light, depend on the sun and the weather.

When the sun is obscured by light cloud the light becomes softer and more diffused. This is ideal light for taking portraits. The intensity of shadows and contrast is reduced. Colour tones are more varied, deeper and richer. You can show subtle details throughout the frame, especially in close-up portraits. If the clouds get heavier, however, the light will become dimmer, reducing the definition in your photographs.

The rising and setting sun projects long shadows that give clear shape and form to things and people. The shadows mark out shapes and this is what professional photographers refer to as 'modelling'. Many people photographers prefer the colour, quality, texture and direction of this light.

Direction

Light can come from any direction and sometimes from more than one direction at the same time. You should ascertain the direction of the light and study the way it falls on your subject. Is it adequate? Does it bring out the features you wish to highlight? If not,

Hindu priest, Singapore

I took the first photograph of this priest while he was standing in the overhead light of the midday sun. His eye sockets are in shadow and so are the areas under his nose and chin. I asked if he would mind stepping into the shade so I could take a better photograph, which he happily did. The light in the second photograph is even and all his facial features are clear. Asking somebody to move slightly can mean the difference between a good and a bad photograph.

◀ 35mm SLR, 85mm lens, 1/125 f8, Ektachrome E100SW

◀◀ 35mm SLR, 85mm lens, 1/125 f4, Ektachrome E100SW

you should move to another position, ask the subject to move to a better location or wait until the clouds move. Directionally, there are four types of light: top lighting, front lighting, back lighting and side lighting.

Top Lighting

Top lighting, when the light hits the subject from directly above, occurs around the middle of the day and makes faces harsh and high-contrasting. If you photograph with top light, look out for shadows under your subject's eyes, nose and chin. The subject's face can also be covered in shadow by the brim of a hat or cap. Two or three hours before or after mid-day, when the sun is not as high in the sky, is a much better time to photograph people, as they can then be lit from the side, back or front.

Front Lighting

Front lighting occurs when the light source is behind the photographer's back. It used to be recommended that photographers stand with the sun over their left shoulder. This dates back to a time when cameras needed all the light they could get for a good exposure. Given the enormous improvements in cameras during the past 50 years, it's completely unnecessary now. In fact, having people look into the light is responsible for numerous poor-quality pictures. People blink, squint or narrow their eyes against the sun, and the shadows falling behind them give the image a flat, uninteresting quality. But front lighting in the early morning or late evening can offer you the opportunity to capture vivid colours.

Miner, Mount Isa, Australia

The sky in outback Australia is sometimes dark blue. In this situation it worked very well, providing a visually strong background to the landscape of this miner.

▲ 35mm SLR, 24mm lens, 1/125 f5.6, Kodachrome 64

Cattle yard, Fitzroy, Australia

Because of the swirling dust particles in the air, the early-morning light is diffused and illuminates parts of the scene in penetrating shafts of light. The dust makes such a picture possible but it can ruin cameras and equipment unless you are careful. I always travel with a small towel that I use for perspiration and keeping dust off my camera gear.

◀ 35mm SLR, 20mm lens, 1/250 f5.6, TRI-X 400

Back Lighting

Back lighting occurs when the light source is behind the subject. If you expose for the back light you will get a silhouette. If you expose for the subject's face and use a flash or reflector to light your subject's face, you will get a halo effect around their head. Back lighting decreases the amount of colour and detail in your photograph but, if handled properly, it can be very dramatic or romantic. Be careful of halation or flare in the lens of the camera. Always use a lens shade when pointing the camera towards the sun or artificial light source.

T'ai chi practice, Hong Kong, China

Victoria Park, Hong Kong, is an exciting place and worth a visit. There is always something happening from sunrise to sunset and interesting pictures are almost guaranteed. Here are two back-lit photographs taken in Victoria Park with different results. In the picture below there is flare because I didn't have a lens shade on the camera and it was aimed directly at the sun. In the second photograph, I used a lens shade and didn't point the camera at the sun.

◀ DSLR, 80-200mm lens at 200mm, 1/800 f6.3, 400 ISO, 2240 x 1488, JPEG, lens shade

▲ DSLR, 80-200mm lens at 200mm, 1/500 f5, 400 ISO, 2240 x 1488, JPEG

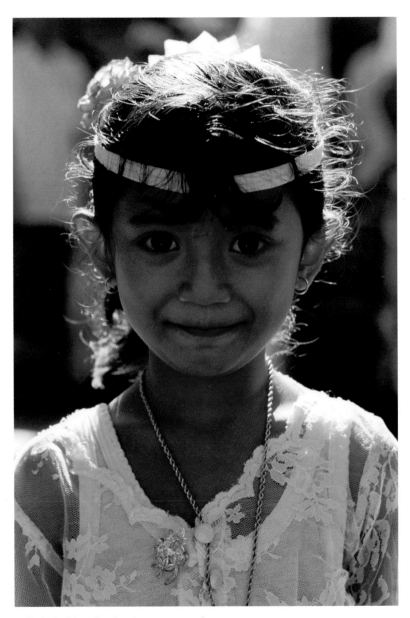

Girl bathed in light, Bali, Indonesia

When wandering around at ceremonies or festivals you'll sometimes come across special moments. I saw this young girl with her family and was immediately struck by the beautiful rim of light that surrounded her head and body.

▲ 35mm SLR, 85mm lens, 1/125 f4, Sensia 100

Outside a teahouse, Isfahan, Iran

Getting up early and going for a walk before breakfast is not only healthy but gives you an opportunity to get early-morning pictures. It was a cold morning when I saw this man waiting outside a teahouse. He nodded at me and I smiled at him as he let me take his photograph. I used a spot meter to expose for the light on his face. The back lighting separated the man from the background.

▲ 35mm SLR, 85mm lens, 1/60 f2.8, Kodachrome 64

Women exercising, Hong Kong, China

Remember that back lighting can be used for groups as well as individuals. The correct skin tones can be achieved by exposing for the light on the faces.

▲ DSLR, 17-35mm lens at 52mm, 1/400 f11, 400 ISO, 3008 x 2000, RAW

Side Lighting

Side lighting occurs when the light source is to the side of the subject. Sunlight around dawn or dusk is a classic example of side lighting, as the sun's rays are entering at an angle from the side. Another instance is window light when the subject stands or sits so that natural light strikes them through a door or window. This sparkling, particle-rich light is wonderful for portraits as it reveals colour and texture. Indeed, it can reveal too much texture – the camera will pick up every wrinkle in the subject's skin.

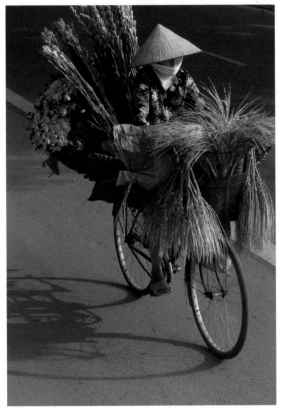

Cyclist in Hanoi, Vietnam

When you first come out of an air-conditioned room or vehicle, remember to give your camera time to adjust to the heat. The first photograph was shot on a hot day straight after the camera was brought out from an air-conditioned room. The lens was fogged by condensation and the exposure is incorrect. The second photograph was taken a short time later, after the camera had adjusted to the ambient temperature.

◀ DSLR, 35-70mm lens at 70mm, 1/200 f11, 200 ISO, 3008 x 2000, RAW, without condensation

▼ DSLR, 35-70mm lens at 35mm, 1/1600 f3.2, 200 ISO, 3008 x 2000, RAW, with condensation

FLASHLIGHT

Flash provides a convenient light source that will let you take a photograph even in the darkest places without having to change films or use a tripod. Most modern compact cameras and SLRs have built-in flash units. Otherwise a separate flash unit can be mounted on the camera via the hot-shoe or off the camera on a flash bracket with a flash lead.

Pictures taken with flash from built-in or hot-shoe mounted units are usually unexceptional. The direct, frontal light is harsh and rarely flattering. It creates hard shadows on surfaces behind the subject and backgrounds are often too dark. To improve the look of your flash photographs, get to know the features of your particular unit. If you have an SLR, explore the possibilities of off-camera flash, bounce flash and fill flash.

Hindu bride with candle, Singapore

The bride is holding a candle in her hands under a canopy in a temple. When photographing indoors, you can expose for the incandescent or artificial light and then use a small amount of flash to fill in the shadows without overpowering the available light.

▲ DSLR, 17-35mm lens at 70mm, 1/10 f3.5, 200 ISO, 2240 x 1488, JPEG

Rice farmer, Bali, Indonesia

I exposed for the background when taking this photo and I also used a flash on a flash lead, with the flash set to underexpose 1/2 a stop so it would light up the man's face. An amber warming filter was attached to the front of the flash, to warm up his face.

◀ 35mm SLR, 35mm lens, 1/125 f8, Ektachrome E100GX

Red-eye

If you use direct, on-camera flash when photographing people, your portraits may suffer from red-eye caused by the flash being in line with the lens and the light reflecting off the blood vessels of the retina straight back onto the film. Red-eye can be minimised with the following techniques:

▸ ask your subject not to look directly into the lens
▸ bounce the flash off a reflective surface
▸ increase the light in the room, so that the subject's pupils close down
▸ move the flash away from the camera lens

Many modern cameras have a red-eye reduction feature, which triggers a short burst of pre-flashes just before the shutter opens. This causes the pupils to close down. It's a sophisticated way of increasing the light in the room.

Off-camera Flash

Off-camera flash gives more pleasing results because the light is moved to the side and above the lens so that it's angled towards the subject. Red-eye is eliminated and shadows fall below the subject, rather than directly behind. A sync lead connects the flash to the camera. You can hold the flash and shoot one-handed, but mounting the flash on a flash bracket makes life a lot easier. Though this will limit the angle you can use, you'll soon be able to anticipate how the flash will light your subject.

Bounce Flash

Even more pleasing results are possible if bounce-flash techniques are employed. You need a flash unit with a tilt head or the ability to mount the flash off-camera on a bracket. The flash is aimed at the ceiling, wall or flash reflector, which bounces the light back at the subject. The light is indirect and soft, and shadows are minimised. However, walls and ceilings come in varying heights and colours and this can present problems. If ceilings are too high you won't be able to bounce the flash. Dark-coloured walls and ceilings will absorb too much of the light. The surface should be white, as coloured surfaces will give your picture a colour cast.

To overcome all these problems a bounce-flash kit is worth the small investment. The flash is bounced off a reflector attached to the flash head, which tilts. The reflectors are interchangeable and available in different colours. A gold reflector will bounce warm light and a silver reflector will bounce cooler light.

Sudanese man, Adelaide, Australia

To capture the warm personality of this man I kept the image very simple and placed him against a plain background. I pointed the flashlight at the white wall to the right of my camera so I had a soft light. The flash picked up the light in his eyes which gave the image a pleasing effect. I used a medium length telephoto lens to keep the picture tight on his face.

◀ 35mm, 85mm lens, 1/125, f5.6, Kodachrome 64 ISO

Rear-curtain Synch

If you set your electronic flash to rear-curtain synch, the flash will fire just before the shutter closes rather than just after it opens. This can result in a stream of light leading to or from your subject if you use a slow shutter speed. If you hold the camera and pan it, this will provide a deliberate blurring effect that likewise takes the viewer's eye to the subject.

Fill Flash

Fill flash is a technique used to add light to shadowed areas containing important detail that would otherwise be rendered too dark. A good example is the use of fill flash to remove shadows from a face. The flash provides a secondary source of light to complement the main light source, usually the sun. If executed well, the flashlight will be unnoticeable, but if it overpowers the main light the photo will look unnatural.

Fill-flash techniques have long been the domain of professional photographers. Now most compact cameras, SLRs with built-in flash units and advanced SLRs with dedicated flash systems have a fill-flash feature. Some activate automatically while others require you to decide that fill flash is needed. Use the fill-flash feature when:

▸ the light on your subject is uneven, such as when a person's hat casts a shadow over their eyes but their nose and mouth are in full sun
▸ your subject is backlit and you don't want to create a silhouette
▸ your subject is in shade, but the background is bright.

Remember, your subject must still be within the effective range of your particular flash unit.

If you're using a less sophisticated SLR and accessory flash, you will need to override the flash so that it delivers less light than it would if it were the main light source (usually one to 1.5 stops less). Set your exposure for the brightest part of your composition, say 1/60 at f8, but set the flash on f5.6 or f4.5. Alternatively, you can change the ISO setting on the flash unit, from say 100 to 200. Both techniques trick the flash into thinking that the scene needs less light than it actually does. Output is reduced, which prevents it becoming the main light source while still giving enough light to fill in the dark areas.

Boat builder, Fremantle, Australia

This man was testing his model boat in the sea. I exposed for the sunset and used a flash unit to fill in the shadows on the man's face and boat. I used a 200mm lens so that I didn't have to stand too close to the spray. If seawater or sand gets into your camera equipment it can cause corrosion very quickly. Use a plastic bag to keep your equipment covered or continually wipe it clean with a cloth covered in WD40.

◀ 35mm SLR, 80-200mm lens at 200mm, 1/125 f4, Kodachrome 64 ISO

INCANDESCENT LIGHT

Incandescent light emanates from floodlights, stage lights, electric light bulbs (incandescent, fluorescent or otherwise), torches, lanterns, candles and, essentially, any form of artificial light.

The points made earlier about the colour, direction and quality of natural light are also relevant to incandescent light. But colour transparency film, if used in non-fluorescent incandescent light, will have a warm orange-yellow tinge or cast. Sometimes this may help capture the mood you're seeking and so you deliberately use daylight transparency film. But often the orange-yellow cast will make your portraits seem surreal, or as if the subject is unwell. You might instead choose to use tungsten transparency film which is balanced for incandescent light. Alternatively, use filters such as an 82A, 82B or 82C, which will remove orange-yellow casts, or an FLD (fluorescent to daylight) filter, which will remove the blue-green cast caused by using colour film balanced for daylight.

Art gallery, Melbourne, Australia

When taking pictures indoors without a flash, try to be aware of the type of lighting that is being used. This art gallery uses fluorescent lighting. The first picture was taken with daylight film. The second picture was also taken with daylight film but a fluorescent filter was used to correct the colour cast. When you use a fluorescent filter you lose a stop of exposure, so you may need to use faster film or a tripod.

◀ 35mm SLR, 24mm zoom lens, 1/4 f4-2.8, Sensia 100, FLD filter, tripod

◀◀ 35mm SLR, 24mm zoom lens, 1/8 f4-2.8, Sensia 100, tripod

Zoroastrian celebrant, Tehran, Iran

I was given permission to enter a temple where a Zoroastrian priest was attending the sacred fires. The incandescent light in the room was combined with window light. This lighting mixture doesn't always work because it's often too warm and turns the skin tone orange. But on this occasion it worked very well because the window light was strong and it helped create a slightly warm but reasonably accurate colour.

◀ 35mm SLR, 24mm lens, 1/30 f2, Kodachrome 64

▸ **When shooting with colour negative film it's not necessary to use correction filters. Colour negative film is designed to be used under most lighting conditions and any corrections that are needed can be made at the printing stage.**

On digital cameras you can change the white-balance settings to suit the type of incandescent light.

In any event, be aware of the contrast range when floodlights, lanterns or candles are the main source of illumination. There can be an enormous range of brightness and intensity between where the light hits the subject and the edge of the lighting, which rapidly falls into shadow. Use the spot meter on your camera, or zoom in on your subject's face, to get an accurate meter reading. If neither of these options is available, bracket your exposures in half-stop increments up to a stop and a half over and under.

Lighting candles, Chinatown, Singapore

This space was lit by hundreds of candles in preparation for a Taoist celebration. Candlelight is always a beautifully warm light by which to photograph. Don't forget that you have to use a tripod, monopod or fast film if you want to pick up details.

◀ 35mm SLR, 85mm lens, 1/15 f2, Sensia 100

PART FOUR:

Human fascination with pictures of others is universal and timeless. Perhaps it's because all people, as soon as they're born, begin studying other people's faces. They continue to do so for the rest of their lives. The choice of whom to photograph when travelling is a reflection of the people photographer's own observations and interests. Certainly there's no shortage of subjects and if it's true that each person has a story worth hearing, then it's equally true each person is a suitable subject for a picture worth seeing.

ON THE ROAD

PORTRAITS

A portrait is a reflective study of a person. A good portrait shows the external appearance of that person and also reveals aspects of his or her character, personality and spirit. The most important aspect on which to concentrate when photographing a portrait is the subject's eyes, so focus on the eyes and expose for the subject's face. Where and how the eyes look is the difference between a mediocre and a good portrait. If you think the face is interesting enough, fill the entire frame with the face.

A person who catches your eye will catch the eye of other people when they look at your photographs, but only if you can show what first drew your eye to that person. It may be the translucent skin of a child or the incredible patchwork of age lines on the face of someone far older. As you approach your subject and work out the composition of your photograph, remember what first attracted your attention. Many times the quality you're after is elusive and cannot be expressed in words. But that quality is what you're aiming to capture visually and it is what you will 'say' in the portrait.

Ideally, spend time with your subject. In practice this is not always possible, especially for a traveller. But initial eye contact and a smile can provide you with a strong sense of a person's personality. Other forms of communication such as words, body language, gestures, jokes or mime will add to your knowledge of your subject. Human beings never cease exchanging signals about themselves, and everything you consciously or intuitively learn about your subject from these brief initial exchanges will feed into the portrait.

Head-hunter, Port Moresby, New Guinea
I was photographing a tour of New Guinea by Pope John Paul II and his large entourage. The yellow and black paint on the face of this man suggested he had prepared for the occasion. Yet, cigarette in lips, he stood aside from the mass of people around the pope. Often the best pictures are captured when you move away from the centre of the action.

▲ 35mm SLR, 85mm lens, 1/125 f4.5, Kodachrome 64

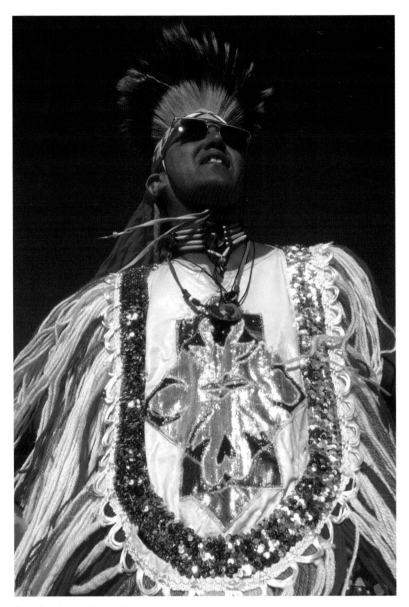

Native American, Las Vegas, USA

Native Americans from all over North America had gathered in Nevada to celebrate their culture and I wanted the picture to do likewise. I photographed this man by lying down on the ground and framing him against the blue sky. The bright colours of his costume glitter in the sunlight.

▲ 35mm SLR, 20mm lens, 1/250 f5.6, Ektachrome E100SW

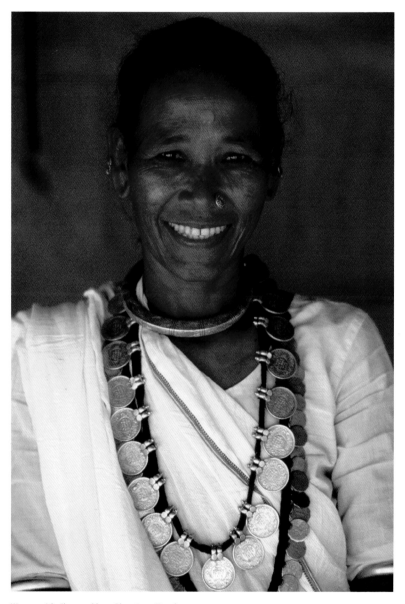

Woman with silver necklace, Bharatpur, Nepal

It was the necklace on this Nepalese woman that first caught my attention. Her pride and good humour were evident in the way she smiled when she saw me. She grinned when I asked if I could photograph her and laughed as I pressed the shutter.

▲ 35mm SLR, 35mm lens, Ektachrome E100SW

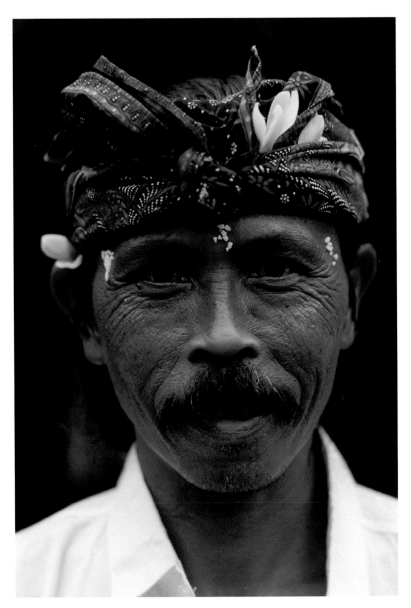

Balinese festival guide, Tampaksiring, Bali, Indonesia

The Balinese are famous for their relaxed charm. This man was busily guiding visitors to a water festival but he paused long enough for me to capture the close-up image that I sought. The diagonal colours of his headscarf help guide the eye to his friendly face.

▲ 35mm SLR, 85mm lens, 1/125 f2.8, Sensia 100

ENVIRONMENTAL PORTRAITS

An environmental portrait frames a person within a setting that reveals or comments on their way of life. For example, additional insight into the life of a carpet weaver or lantern-maker can be shown by including part of their workplace. Or an environmental portrait of a person in traditional costume at an age-old festival engaged in a cellphone conversation can make its own comment on the juxtaposition of modern life and traditional culture. Essentially, environmental portraits allow you to explore how and where people fit, or sometimes don't fit, in their world.

Environmental portraits do not have the same intimacy as close-ups where the subject fills the frame, but they do provide additional valuable information. Indeed, the viewer will sometimes find it difficult to relate to the people in your photographs without knowing their social or occupational context. Including the environment can above all enhance your ability to look into the subject's life, to hint at how they themselves might see the world.

Be careful not to include so much of the environment that the subject is lost and occupies only an insignificant proportion of the image. A successful environmental portrait creates a dynamic balance between the person and their environment.

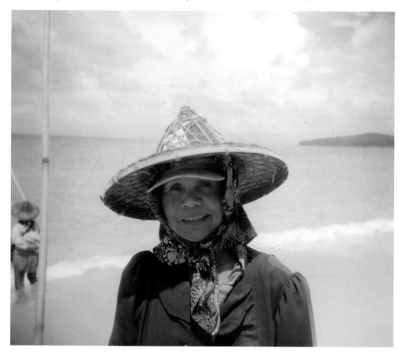

Fisherwoman, Phuket, Thailand

This fisherwoman spends a lot of time on the beach, fishing in the serene calm. My plastic Holga point-and-shoot camera seemed the best way to capture her ethereal quality.

▲ Holga 120, Fujicolor NPC 160

Snake man, Renmark, Australia

Personally, I dislike snakes. But the subject was a snake expert so it seemed natural to photograph him with two of the pythons from his collection of more than 200 reptiles. I used a bounce flash to soften the lighting. I also adjusted the aperture so the background was exposed slightly darker than the snake expert.

▲ 35mm SLR, 35mm lens, 1/60 f8, Kodachrome 64

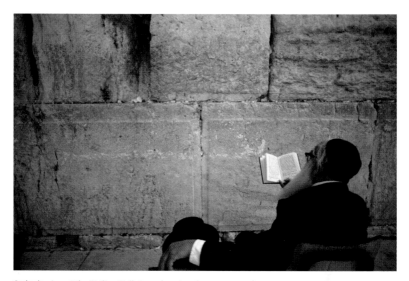

Orthodox Jew at the Wailing Wall, Jerusalem, Israel

This gentleman reading his prayers was oblivious to my presence. The white page of his prayer book reflects light back on his face and is offset by his white shirt cuff.

▲ 35mm SLR, 20mm lens, 1/125 f4, Kodachrome 64

Silat swordsman, Brisbane, Australia

This man was practising the Indonesian sport of Silat in a park. When photographing any sport, try to follow the athlete with your camera and anticipate action.

▲ 35mm SLR, 20mm lens, 1/250 f4, Kodachrome 64

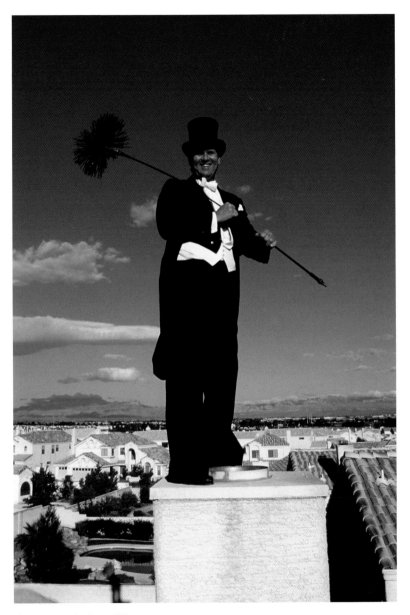

Chimney sweep, Las Vegas, USA

Despite his immaculate top hat and tails, this man is a genuine chimney sweep. I met him when I was on assignment in Las Vegas and he invited me to join him at his current workplace.

▲ 35mm SLR, 35-70mm lens at 35mm, 1/125 f5.6, Ektachrome E100SW

GROUPS

Group portraits can provide wonderful insights into how people relate to each other on an everyday basis. Social and gregarious by nature, people will gather together for dozens of reasons. Certainly the sight of a foreigner with a camera often seems to be a good enough cause. Given the random nature of travelling, the social gatherings you come upon are likely to be casual rather than formal. Whatever the reason for the gathering, it's sure to be entertaining.

Composition becomes challenging when photographing groups. You must design a picture with people. Usually this means asking them to shift around until you're satisfied with the final configuration. Sometimes you'll wish to make a particular person more dominant, or at least establish his or her relationship with the group. Stairways, garden walls, slopes and inclines allow you to place people on different levels. You might well find somewhere higher to shoot from. You don't want one person or their shadow to be obscuring another person but neither do you want the group to be too dispersed. Take several shots. The larger the group, the greater the likelihood that someone has blinked or looked away as you released the shutter.

When using a wide-angle lens (24mm or shorter), be aware that it might distort the people on the edge of the frame.

If you're trying to photograph an individual who is part of a group, it's advisable to photograph the group first. You can then ask the people to step aside from the individual whose portrait you wish to make, or move closer or zoom in on the individual.

Afternoon tea, Napier, New Zealand

The town of Napier is one of the major Art Deco centres of the world. Local people were enjoying a 1930s dress-up party when I visited. I shot from down low and used a wide-angle lens to capture the different characters.

▲ 35mm SLR, 20mm lens, 1/125 f2.8, Ektachrome E100SW

Orthodox Christian pilgrims, Jerusalem, Israel

Huge crowds of pilgrims packed Jerusalem for Greek Orthodox Easter on an extremely hot day. The streets were full of processions, cymbals were sounding and the air was full of incense. These celebrants had found some shade for a temporary rest. Sometimes a group rather than a crowd gives a lasting sense of occasion.

▲ 35mm SLR, 35mm lens, 1/60 f4, Ektachrome E100SW

Boys in uniform, Suai, East Timor

Sometimes you might photograph a group of people because of their geometry. The scarves, shirts and braces of these uniformed boys were all in a V shape. Even the way they stood formed a V.

▲ 35mm SLR, 35mm lens, 1/250 f11, TRI-X 400

CROWDS

Crowds come in all shapes and sizes, and they can vary in purpose, character and mood just like individuals. Crowds might consist of revellers dancing at Mardi Gras, a cheering mass of supporters at a sporting event, worshippers congregating at a religious festival, eager bargain-hunters at a market or the crowds of commuters who pack the streets and subways of any major city early and late in the day.

Often the challenge is to find a way to show the crowd as something more than a shapeless mass of anonymity. Look for ways to break up the crowd or to mark out individuals. It also helps to photograph a section of the crowd that best represents or symbolises the event you are witnessing.

Food stalls, Singapore

This market was lit by a mixture of incandescent, fluorescent and tungsten lights, creating many different colour casts. I used colour negative film because it is much easier to control than slide film during the printing process. I stood on a large box so I could shoot over the crowd.

▲ 35mm SLR, 20mm lens, 1/4 f5.6, Fijicolor NPH 400, tripod

Monks, Angkor Wat, Cambodia

There was a huge crowd of visitors at Angkor Wat. The best way to isolate these monks was for me to lie down and photograph the colours of their robes against the blue sky.

▲ 35mm SLR, 20mm lens, 1/60 f4, Ektachrome E100SW

Women Praying, Singapore

A good way to illustrate what is going on in a large crowd is to concentrate on a small section. I knelt down on the floor and shot between the rows of people so I could isolate these women and capture a picture of them praying.

▲ DSLR, 17-35mm lens at 25mm, 1/250 f5, 200 ISO, 3008 x 2000, RAW

Crowd at the Wailing Wall, Jerusalem, Israel

So much is always happening in a crowd. Groups form and reform in separate cameos. The secret is to watch and wait until the composition feels right.

▲ 35mm SLR, 20mm lens, 1/250 f4, Ektachrome E100SW

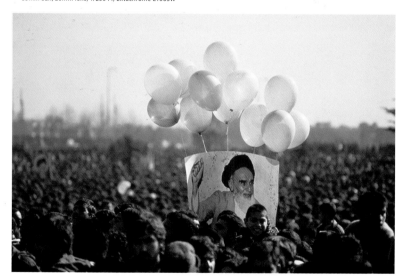

Anniversary of the founding of the Republic of Iran.

When photographing large crowds, it's wise to have at least two zoom lenses to choose from. Two million people were on the streets of Tehran to celebrate the founding of the Republic of Iran. After I took the photograph, a companion lifted me up and I literally ran across the top of the crowd to escape the exuberance of the people.

▲ 35mm SLR, 300mm lens, 1/250 f4, Kodachrome 64

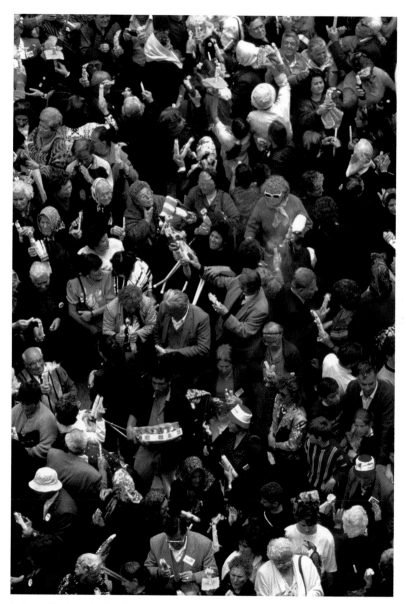

Easter candles, Jerusalem, Israel

Seek out a high vantage point when photographing a crowd, for it allows you many options. For example, you can use a long lens to focus in on different sections of the crowd or even individual faces. Alternatively, a wide-angle shot can show the crowd milling around.

▲ 35mm SLR, 20mm lens, 1/250 f8, Ektachrome E100SW

CHILDREN

Children are the centre of attention in many images. They're usually less nervous and more enthusiastic about being photographed than adults. They're also unpredictable and chameleon-like. They will almost inevitably surprise you with a new expression or a new physical antic, even as you prepare to press the shutter release. If they become overexcited, trying to photograph them is like trying to shepherd fish. Nevertheless, they are superb photographic subjects. Be ready to shoot fast, and often, as their changes of expression are so many, and so fleeting.

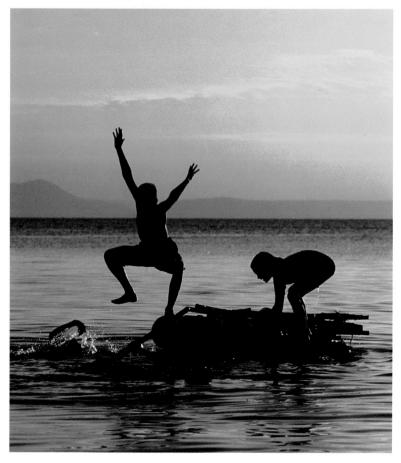

Boys leaping from raft, Lake Taupo, New Zealand

With a long lens I was able to silhouette these children against the setting sun. Whenever you're photographing on the beach be careful not to let sand get into your camera gear. After I have been working at the beach I always use a blower brush to clean my equipment.

▲ 35mm SLR, 80-200mm lens at 200mm, 1/250 f8, Ektachrome E100SW

Sisters in the temple, Singapore

Never be afraid to ask people if they would like to be photographed. The parents of these children were very proud when I took this picture.

▲ 35mm SLR, 35mm lens, 1/60 f2, Ektachrome E100SW

Father, son and toy cat, Las Vegas, USA

I spent a lot of time at this Native American festival, wandering around the perimeters, and was rewarded with this image. The sleeping child was holding the toy with the same affection as the father was holding the child, and it was this that first caught my eye.

▲ 35mm SLR, 24mm lens, 1/125 f4, Ektachrome E100SW

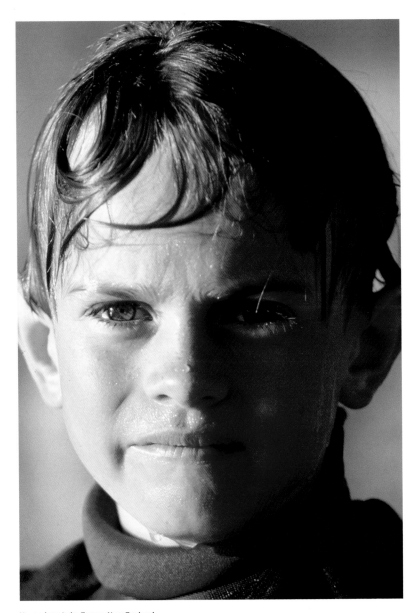

Young boy, Lake Taupo, New Zealand

This boy has just climbed out of the lake and there is water still dripping from his face. Gazing back at his friends, he is unaware of the camera as I used a long lens. Sometimes it is a good idea to use a long lens to capture candid pictures, especially with children, who often pose if they realise they're being photographed.

▲ 35mm SLR, 80-200mm lens, 1/500 f4.5, Ektachrome E100SW

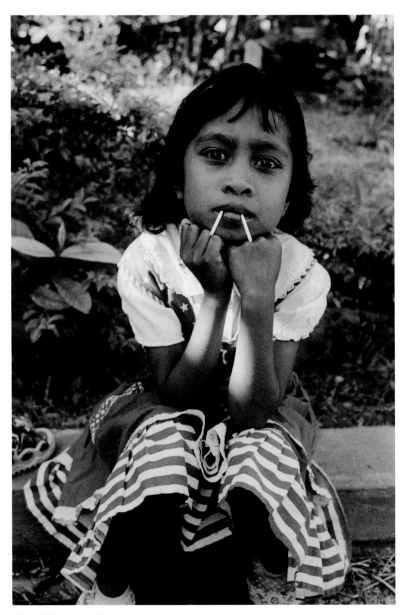

Girl with lollipops, Suai, East Timor

I saw this girl with two lollipops in her mouth out of the corner of my eye. Remember that what catches your eye will catch the eye of others.

▲ 35mm SLR, 35mm lens, 1/500 f8, TRI-X 400

TRAVEL COMPANIONS

The people you share your travels with will probably be some of your most photographed subjects. Indeed, travellers often return with a sort of miniseries of images of their companions. These pictures work best when they show their friends in new and unusual places. Photograph your companions with the same care and inspiration you bring to the photography of anyone else.

Photographers photographing photographers, Singapore

I was photographing the Singapore skyline when I saw these tourists taking pictures of each other. When taking pictures of your companions remember to include some of the surroundings.

◀ 35mm SLR, 20mm lens, 1/250 f5.6, Ektachrome E100SW

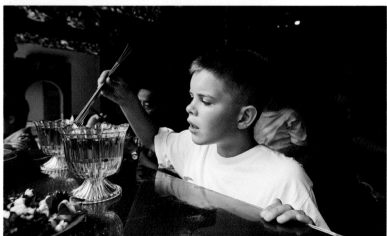

Western boy with incense, Chinatown, Singapore

When travelling with companions, try to photograph them in environments that reflect the variety of places visited. In this Chinese temple, I waited until the boy turned his face to the daylight and lit the incense. I exposed for the light on his face, allowing the temple to go into comparative darkness.

▲ 35mm SLR, 20mm lens, 1/250 f2.8, Fujicolor 400 ISO

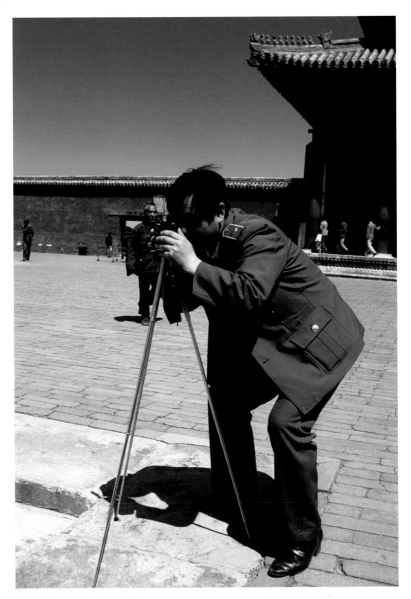

Family photographer, Beijing, China

The man photographing his family is shooting in bright sunlight. The correct exposure in such circumstances would be f16 with the shutter speed set at the ISO of his film. The most advisable shutter speed for an ISO film of 100 in bright sunlight is 1/100, for an ISO of 400 the shutter speed should be 1/400 (or the nearest shutter speed, which is 1/500).

▲ 35mm SLR, 20mm lens, Kodachrome 64

LOW LIGHT

Photographing people in low light is a challenge that can be met in several ways. Some of the best and most famous photographs of people have been taken in low light. With the equipment and high-speed film available today it's true that if you can see it, you can photograph it. Dramatic pictures of people outdoors in bad weather conditions presuppose low light as do softer images of people in snow, mist or rain, and many night-time photographs of people indoors. In low-light conditions it's almost certainly necessary to use a fast to very fast film (200 ISO to 1000 ISO) or to set your digital camera to a higher than normal ISO setting. A fast film or sensor setting also means you may be able to select smaller apertures for greater depth of field, as well as faster shutter speeds for subjects in motion.

Alternatively, you can shoot on a slow shutter speed with your camera mounted on a tripod or monopod to avoid camera shake. This should only be done when your subject is not likely to move and when you can be sure there will be no other form of visual interference whilst the shutter is open. Avoid shutter speeds slower than 1/8 of a second as the chances of camera or subject movement will be high.

Flash provides a third option for dealing with low light. However, over-flashing can reduce or remove the ambient atmosphere you may be trying to capture. So be careful about how much flash you put into the picture. Use it only as a fill and not as the main source of light.

If you're shooting in low light with a compact camera, and you've turned off the flash, it's best to compose your picture with the zoom lens set at the wide-angle position rather than the telephoto position. The wide-angle option on most compact cameras lets in four times more light, which increases the chance of successfully hand-holding the camera.

Tailors, Dubai

These tailors were working inside a bazaar. There were already other pictures exposed on the roll of film I had in the camera, so I couldn't push the film to a higher ISO. I turned the shutter speed to a 1/8 of a second, rested firmly against a wall and waited until I was breathing very calmly to minimise the risk of camera shake.

▲ 35mm SLR, 20mm lens, 1/8 f2, Kodachrome 64

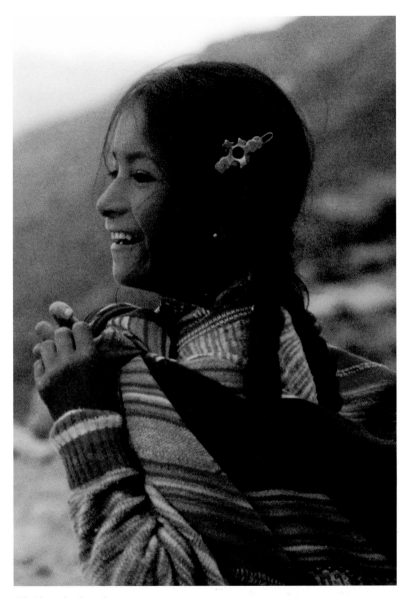

Girl with poncho, Cuzco, Peru

Never miss an opportunity. Early one evening our car broke down in the Andes. I'm not much of a mechanic so while my companions fixed our vehicle I wandered off taking pictures. I spotted this girl as she walked along a dirt track from her village through the hills. There was just enough light to capture her image as she disappeared down the mountainside.

▲ 35mm SLR, 35mm lens, 1/125 f4, Agfa 400

Fish sellers with customers, Hong Kong, China

Inside the early-morning fish market, the light was low. Rather than use a flash, I pushed the ISO of the film up two stops, from 200 to 800 ISO. Pushing up the ISO to a higher number is often a good option when working in low light.

▲ 35mm SLR, 85mm lens, 1/125 f2.8, Ektachrome E200 pushed two stops to 800 ISO

Chinese opera singers, Singapore

These Chinese opera singers are waiting in the backstage area before their performance. When shooting in low light with a digital camera, you can switch the ISO up to a higher number, in this case to 800 ISO. Don't forget to change the white balance if the lighting is fluorescent.

▲ DSLR, 17-35mm lens at 19mm, 1/8 f2.8, 400 ISO, 2240 x 1488, JPEG

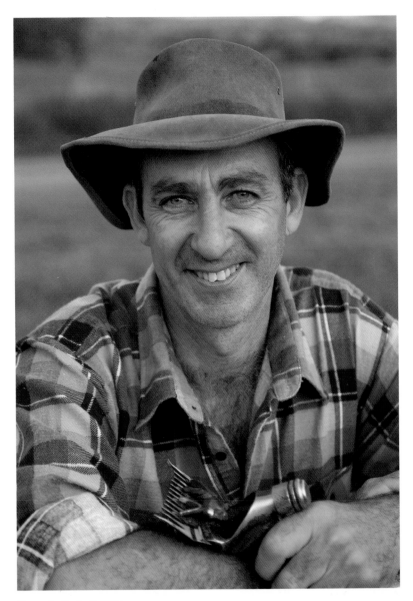

Shearer, Heathcote, Australia

It was late in afternoon when I saw this man leaning on a fence in the Australian countryside talking to his friends. The light was very low and the hat cast a shadow over his eyes. I asked him to tilt his hat back to get rid of the shadow. Then one of his friends held a reflector next to the camera which brightened up his face and added a sparkle to his eyes. By simply including this man's tools of trade, the comb, he is identified as a shearer.

▲ DSLR, 35-70mm lens at 52mm, 1/200 F3.2, 200 ISO, 3008 x 2000, RAW

INDOORS

Photographing people indoors can result in pictures equally as appealing as those of people outdoors. Homes, workplaces, shops, restaurants, hotels, galleries, museums, temples and churches are only some of the varied indoor places where people photographers can take great pictures. However, in some of them, especially in places of art and religion, flashlights, tripods and monopods are often not permitted. Prior permission to take photographs and/or the payment of a fee may also be required. Don't let this stop you from seeking out people within such places.

▸ **Natural light, indoors, can be entrancing. Positioning people near a window or doorway provides plentiful opportunities for beautifully lit images. This type of light is a favourite with many photographers and they often seek to reproduce it in studio portraits.**

Incandescent or low light indoors presents various challenges and opportunities, as previously discussed. Additionally, if you're photographing someone indoors, you might see if you can obtain permission to shift some of the light sources around if it's absolutely vital to use a particular location. It's much easier to ask your subject to move to a better lit part of the room or building. When taking candid photographs you'll have to wait for the subject to move into such an area. If a particular place within the building is important, and is well lit, then prepare your camera settings for that space and wait for a suitable person to come along.

Women window-shopping for jewellery, Tehran, Iran

I took this picture from inside, shooting out through the shop window. I took a spot meter reading of the jewellery before there was anybody there. Then I waited until some ladies who were window-shopping stopped to look at the jewellery.

▲ 35mm SLR, 24mm lens, 1/125 f2.8, Kodachrome 64

Muslim woman, Marawi, Philippines

This woman is close to the window and is turned at a three-quarter view so that the light covers most of her body and face.

▲ 35mm SLR, 24mm lens, 1/30 f2.8, Kodachrome 64

Monk, Siem Riep, Cambodia

The window light on the monk falls only on his face and shoulders. This is because he is directly in front of the window and facing it. The rest of his body is in shadow because the walls behind him are too dark to reflect the window light.

▲ 35mm SLR, 35mm lens, 1/15 f2, Sensia 100

ON THE STREET

On the passing pageant of the streets, a million wonderful moments happen every day. A begging monk in a saffron robe may be silhouetted for an instant against a dawn sky, young boys may kick a football as they make their way to school, a street barber may be cutting the hair of a customer, or a woman wearing a conical hat and laden down with fresh vegetables may pass by on her bicycle. You might find all this and much more in a new country, especially during those first days when your eyes are still fresh. Local people grow so accustomed to their world that they don't see it in the same way you do.

Sometimes you might spot a wonderful background such as a poster-decorated wall, a street corner or, often, the doorways and entrances to the worlds off the street. It pays then to sit opposite the location (a café isn't a bad choice) whilst you watch and wait for the right person to come along. Perseverance is a quality that all good photographers should have. They also need the patience to wait until the light is right and have the good sense to go somewhere else if the photo opportunity is not going to happen.

Anticipation is the key to street photography. Observe people and try to anticipate if they're heading into a place or position that will be interesting, quirky or entertaining. At such times, find the best location and wait for them to appear in the frame. There are few things more frustrating than to see a magic moment and then to realise it has passed before you can raise the camera to your eye. But unless you can anticipate what is going to happen, you will not be ready with your camera.

Cleaning woman, Las Vegas, USA

Las Vegas is a night-time city but it is the behind-the-scenes people who can provide the most telling images. Shortly after dawn, the only person on an entire avenue of casinos was this cleaning woman. I placed myself in a position where I thought the background was interesting and waited until the woman appeared.

▲ 35mm SLR, 20mm lens, 1/125 f5.6, Ektachrome E100SW

Three bridesmaids, Siem Riep, Cambodia

I watched patiently until these bridesmaids' bodies, faces and umbrellas formed an interesting composition.

▲ 35mm SLR, 24mm lens, 1/125 f4, Sensia 100

Boy on bicycle, Dili, East Timor

I visited this area in the early morning on a number of occasions because I liked the way the light was shinning on the road and the way it backlit the palm trees. I sat on a rock and watched and waited for something to happen. I saw this cyclist in the distance and followed him in the viewfinder waiting until he was positioned between the trees with his shadow stretching along the road. This image is about the essentials of photography, shape and form, light and shadow.

▲ 35mm SLR, 35mm lens, 1/500 f8, Kodak TRIX 400

PARKS & GARDENS

Public parks and gardens are great places for photographing people. You'll see them sleeping, picnicking, promenading, strolling, jogging, running, horse-riding, skateboarding and roller-skating. They ice-skate on frozen lakes in winter and sunbathe in summer. They feed birds, fish and eels. They practise t'ai chi. They rehearse and perform dances and practise with musical instruments. Buskers and jugglers often entertain. Make sure you watch the people being entertained – often they make better subjects than the entertainer.

Picnic in the park, Napier, New Zealand

This couple were having their own private little festival during a much larger festival of 1930s Art Deco. It was a cold, cloudy day so I used an 81A warming filter to slightly brighten up the colours.

◀ 35mm SLR, 20mm lens, 1/125 f4, Ektachrome E100SW

Picnic in the park, Tehran, Iran

Tehran is a pleasant city with many parks full of people during the holidays and warmer weather. One afternoon I was strolling through a park in the centre of the city when I saw this man lying on a rug as his family packed away the picnic articles. His face broke into a grin when I pointed the camera at him and he nodded in agreement, allowing me to take his picture.

▲ 35mm SLR, 24mm lens, 1/125 f4, Kodachrome 64

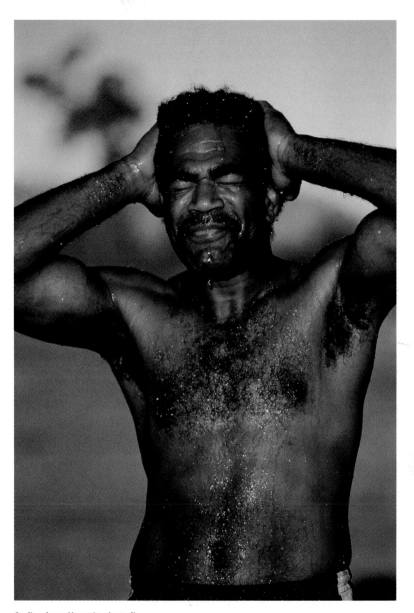

Cooling down, Mount Isa, Australia

This athlete had exercised vigorously during the afternoon heat in a Mount Isa park in the northern part of Australia. I watched him as he stood under a tap and sprayed water over himself to cool down. He stood there meditating as I shot a few frames of cooling water and his own perspiration trickling down his body.

▲ 35mm SLR, 80-200mm lens at 200mm, 1/500 f2.8, Kodachrome 64

MARKETS

All marketplaces are different but essentially it's the people in the market who make the difference. Roaming a market guarantees you'll come across unique characters. The vendors and the buyers present extraordinary opportunities for wonderful visual compositions made from clothes, body shapes and faces. People are alert but often too busy with their transactions to take more than a passing interest in a foreigner's camera. The diversity of stalls means there are many different backgrounds, foregrounds and framing configurations available.

Town markets are at their busiest in the early morning, when the sun's beautiful light is a soft orange, yellow or red. The morning shadows are long and physical definitions are clear. However, many stall owners put up heavy shade cloths to protect their goods from the sun. It is sometimes necessary to use flash to cope with the shadowy interiors dappled with shafts of light. Roofed markets are often dimly lit by fluorescent tubes or tungsten lights, so all your low-light photography skills will be needed.

City markets are usually open every day but small town and village markets are often held on a weekly or even monthly basis. These tend to be festive events with entertainers, and local people rather than professional market vendors selling goods. Art-and-craft markets also bring out artists and locals. All are happy hunting grounds for photographers looking for people in interesting settings.

Market vendor, Hong Kong, China

When shooting with a slow shutter speed and a flash, it's important to look for a background that allows the subject to stand out.

◀ 35mm SLR, 24mm lens, 1/15 f4, Sensia 100, flash with rear-curtain sync

Clothes market, Dili, East Timor

Business was quiet and this vendor was resting when I arrived at the market. His friend turned around to check out the camera. Just as he turned I pressed the shutter and because his face was so close to the lens it created a three-dimensional effect.

◀ 35mm SLR, 20mm lens, 1/250 f8, TRI-X 400

Hammering the metal, Shiraz, Iran

Shafts of window light can be used to make beautiful photographs. I asked this man to shift around slightly until the shaft of light fell directly onto his hammer.

▲ 35mm SLR, 35mm lens, 1/15 f5.6, Kodachrome 64

FESTIVALS

Colourful and dynamic festivals offer superb opportunities for photography. People at festivals are often friendly, helpful and agreeable to having their photograph taken. All sorts of people appear in bright costumes, people whom you otherwise might never get to see. You can often move in quite close and shoot interesting pictures with wide-angle lenses as long as you're not interfering in someone's fun. Move in close to musical instruments such as brass tubas, for example, and you're likely to find reflections in the instrument of the musician, the crowd or the festival. A high vantage point will allow you to photograph the crowd. Try to capture the whole occasion – the mood and crowds with wide shots, as well as full lengths and portraits that, when combined, tell the story of the festival.

Hindu festival, Singapore

During the Hindu Thaipussam festival, celebrants pierce their body and carry milk from temple to temple. There is always the temptation to be aloof and to step back, but in my experience it's better to step forwards. Get involved and get close to the action.

◀ 35mm SLR, 20mm lens, 1/250 f4, Ektachrome E100SW

Drummers, Mt Hagen, New Guinea

Every picture is a record of the interaction between the photographer and the subject. In this case the drummers were in a world of their own as they performed at a highland festival.

◀ 35mm SLR, 24mm lens, 1/250 f4, Kodachrome 64

Ngenteg Linggih festival, Bali, Indonesia

Whenever I'm working at a festival I try to get there early so I can check out the location and hopefully get pictures of entertainers getting ready or rehearsing. At this festival I became so involved with the images that I suddenly found myself standing in the middle of the stage during a performance! A festival gives you the opportunity to make a small picture story: preparing for the show, rehearsing and performing.

◀ 35mm SLR, 85mm lens, 1/60 f4, Sensia 200

◀ 35mm SLR, 24mm lens, 1/60 f4, Sensia 200

▶ 35mm SLR, 85mm lens, 1/60 f4, Sensia 200

▼ 35mm SLR, 85mm lens, 1/125 f4, Sensia 200

PARADES & PROCESSIONS

Parades and processions that form part of people's ceremonies, rituals and celebrations cry out to be captured by the camera. Position is everything in these situations. Look for a high vantage point such as a hill or the upper levels of a multistorey car park. Ideally, if you're going to photograph a parade or procession, travel the route the day before. Look for the vantage points and work out where the light is going to be coming from and what sort of backgrounds you'll have. Also make sure that your most treasured position isn't going to be roped off for dignitaries.

If you can't reconnoitre early and arrange things beforehand, then you're probably going to be restricted to a spot with limited possibilities whilst the procession moves past. The press of the crowd or the need to stay with travelling companions will probably also limit your movement. So, if you can arrange it, bring along a box or metal container to stand on, or even borrow a small ladder. This will help you get a better viewpoint and enable you to shoot over the heads of the crowd. Alternatively, see if you can gain entry to a hotel balcony or a room with an open window overlooking the parade route. Local people watching the parade on balconies are often very sympathetic to the needs of a photographer, and shopkeepers are usually not averse to people entering their premises.

If you use a long lens from above the crowd you will find that the lens gives a telescopic effect by compressing everything. If you shoot with a wide-angle lens from above, you have the opportunity to photograph the procession and also show the surrounding environment, be it a village street, town square or cityscape. If you choose to join the parade, and move along with it, you will probably be free to photograph the marchers from as many angles and with as many different backgrounds as you wish. This usually depends on obtaining prior permission and being careful, for your own and others' safety, to not get in the way of the people in the parade.

The starting and finishing areas of the parade are also worth visiting. At those points people are gathered around, wearing their costumes. They're usually delighted to be photographed and will often pose for your camera.

Buckingham Palace, London, England

The strong reds of the jackets and the shadow bars between the soldiers enliven this picture. I used a long lens and shot down the line for a symmetrical pattern. The rails at Buckingham Palace were handy, as I could put the camera through the bars and then lean against them to remain steady while photographing.

◀ 35mm SLR, 80-200mm lens at 200mm, 1/250 f5.6, Sensia 100

Soldiers marching, Tehran, Iran

When taking travel pictures you need to be prepared to change your plans. I intended to take photographs of these soldiers from the side of the road until I saw how high they were lifting their legs. I lay down in the middle of the road so I could catch the peak of the action as they marched over the top of me.

▲ 35mm SLR, 20mm lens, 1/124 f5.6, Kodachrome 64

Musician, New Delhi, India

There were thousands of people in a procession celebrating Indian Independence Day. I crouched down and shot upwards, framing this musician against the sky to isolate him from the crowd.

▲ 35mm SLR, 20mm lens, 1/250 f5.6, Ektachrome E100SW

ON STAGE

Actors, dancers, singers, musicians and other performers are fascinating to photograph, and they are usually unique to each country. On stage they can be both themselves and not themselves as they represent a different character and role. Furthermore, their costumes and movements can be colourful and exuberant. However, theatres, concert halls and performance spaces are normally lit by tungsten stage lights. So, if you're shooting colour slide film, use tungsten-balanced film or a colour-correction filter – stage lights are normally very warm and produce an orange colour cast on daylight-balanced film.

Stage lights can also change colour at the press of a technician's finger. Equally as quickly, they can fade away to almost nothing and then blaze up again with the entry of a new stage character or the introduction of a fresh choreographic movement. If the people you wish to photograph, or aspects of the performance, are very important to you, then see a performance beforehand. You can then anticipate what is going to happen on stage when you return for the photo shoot. For most travellers, though, this is neither practical nor economical. The main thing is to stay alert so that you're ready for sudden changes in light and movement.

Spot-metering your subject is advisable as a general light reading could result in under- or overexposed sections of a stage that is lit by a variety of lights. Taking a reading of the light falling on a dancer under a spotlight, for example, means you don't have to worry about the lights elsewhere.

An 80-200mm zoom lens is ideal as it gives you the ability to fill the frame with individual performers from your position in the audience. Your position can be improved if you get permission to photograph from the side. When shooting from the audience the use of fast film such as 200 or 400 ISO is very helpful and gives you more options to get better pictures.

If you want to illustrate the action on stage, try shooting with a slow shutter speed to capture blur and swirling colour. Shutter speeds between 1/15 and 1/4 of a second will give you a pleasing result, but shoot lots of frames to be sure. You'll need to use a tripod or monopod to prevent camera shake, or you can rest a small table-top tripod on your chest if you have a seat with a clear view. Placing your camera on a bag or backpack can be almost as effective.

Concert, Dili, East Timor

There were 25,000 people at this concert in a sports stadium. I purposely blurred the picture to convey the dynamics of the night, especially the on-stage energy of the musicians. Don't be afraid to experiment and break the rules of photography. You'll often surprise yourself with the creative images you can achieve.

◀ 35mm SLR, 24mm lens, 1/8 f5.6, TRI-X 400

Nightclub, Mexico City, Mexico

The best angle in a nightclub is one from which you can include both the performers and patrons. The face of the man in the front row as he studies the singer is what makes this picture work.

▲ 35mm SLR, 24mm lens, 1/30 f2.8, Ektachrome EPH 400

Chinese opera performers, Singapore

Stage lights are usually tungsten lights, so it's best to use tungsten film or switch your digital camera to tungsten. If possible, use a tripod or monopod so you can steady the camera as you shoot. With a zoom lens you have the option of photographing the whole stage or, alternatively, getting close-ups of the performers.

▲ DSLR, 35-70mm lens at 55mm, 1/250 f3.2, 800 ISO, 3008 x 2000, RAW

SILHOUETTES

A silhouette occurs when the light behind the subject is brighter than the subject. To create a silhouette, expose for the bright background. The greater the contrast between the subject and the background, the greater the effect. Silhouetting people entails a loss of detail but the resulting image can be striking as it is imbued with depth and dramatic impact. Composition is critical, as the elements within the frame must be separated to ensure the outline of the subject is not lost in darkness or overwhelmed by the intensity of the back light.

It's important not to point your lens at the source of light (eg the sun) because it will create flare in the lens. Try to keep your subject between the camera and the light source.

Fisherman, Hamilton Island, Australia

A dramatically lit image can be obtained by placing the subject in line with the setting sun and its reflection in the water.

◀ 35mm SLR, 24mm lens, 1/60 f4, Ektachrome E100SW

Falconer, Dubai

Always expect the unexpected and move fast when it happens. One afternoon when I was travelling across the desert to photograph some sheiks, I saw this falconer framed against the sky. I stopped the jeep and ran across the desert just in time to take the photo before the sun set.

▲ 35mm SLR, 80-200mm lens at 200mm, 1/250 f4, Ektachrome E100SW

Stockman with dog, Mia Mia, Australia

While I was taking their photograph the stockman and his dog both became interested in something on the distant horizon. Their profiles added extra interest to the image.

▲ 35mm SLR, 80-200mm lens at 200mm, 1/250 f2.8, Ektachrome E100SW

ACTION

The best techniques for photographing people in motion are freezing the action, blur and panning with the camera. Action photographs are essentially dynamic. For example, there might be a colourful swirl of a bullfighter's cape in a blur of movement. A female dancer might seem to defy gravity as she remains frozen in space or floats through the air. The moment a tennis racquet makes contact with the ball might be frozen, or there might be a blur as the ball passes by.

Bullfighter, Mexico City, Mexico

Though the action is blurred, you can still see the eye of the bullfighter. At the height of the action there is always a still point and that is the ideal time to hit the shutter release.

◀ 35mm SLR, 300mm lens, 1/15 f11, Kodachrome 64

Freezing the Action

Any human action can be frozen in great detail by using a fast shutter speed. The actual speed selected will depend on the swiftness of the movement. If someone is running towards you then you can use 1/125 of a second, but if they're running past you a speed of 1/250 or higher is necessary. Outdoors, 100 ISO film is usually satisfactory but on a day with heavy cloud, and indoors, you need to change up to 400 or 800 ISO film or the equivalent sensor setting. Fast shutter speeds mean wider apertures and less depth of field. Careful focussing is vitally important, especially when using a telephoto lens.

Gridiron players, Corvalis, USA

I photographed these gridiron players during their warm-ups because I thought it was just as interesting as the actual game.

◀ 35mm SLR, 135mm lens, 1/250 f4, Kodachrome 64

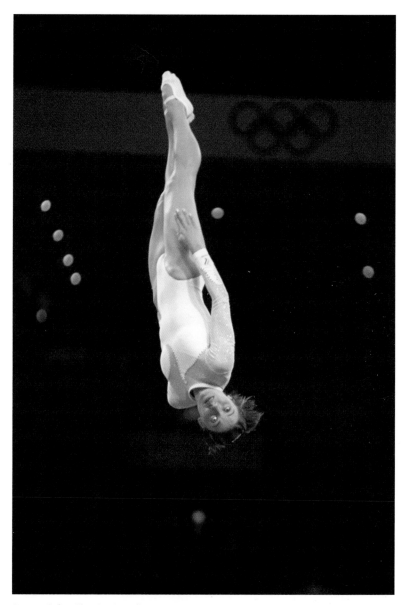

Gymnast, Sydney Olympics, Australia

I had been watching the athletes perform for some time so I knew what they were attempting to do. As this woman left the ground I followed her in the viewfinder of my camera. When she started her routine I kept my finger on the motor drive until she passed through the peak of the performance.

▲ 35mm SLR, 80-200mm lens at 200mm, 1/250 f2.8, Kodak Supra 800

Panning

Panning consists of moving the camera with the subject and releasing the shutter as the subject passes by. Keep moving the camera for a moment afterwards in order to achieve an even swing. Do not move your feet or use jerky body movements. A smooth pan is most productively achieved when you swivel from the hips and swing your entire upper torso. Panning is used to convey a strong impression of movement by keeping the subject in sharp detail against a blurred background. As with freezing the action, the shutter speed you select will depend on the speed of the subject's movement. Generally, shutter speeds of 1/60, 1/30 or 1/15 of a second will give you good results.

Horse-rider, Mansfield, Australia

When panning action pictures you must keep the lower part of your body still and move the camera along with the subject. Press the shutter as the subject goes past but keep moving the camera to get a smooth pass.

▲ 35mm SLR, 35-70mm lens at 70mm, 1/30 f8, Kodachrome 64

Blurring

Blurring emphasises movement by holding the camera still and allowing the subject to move during the exposure. You can achieve it by hand-holding the camera if the subject is moving reasonably quickly or by using a monopod or tripod. Use a slow shutter speed, somewhere between 1/4 and 1/60 of a second. The result can be subtle or bold. It's possible to blur the person in motion and/or whatever else is moving. If you wish the person to remain sharp against a moving background, ask them not to move or wait for a pause in their movement. Everything else moving in the frame will be blurred. Occasionally you can blur everything and create an impressionistic or abstract effect by slightly moving the camera. Indeed this combination of blurring and panning is one of the ways you can experiment and further your knowledge of what imaginative photography can achieve. You might also try releasing the shutter as you zoom in or out with a zoom lens. This changes the focal length during the exposure and produces a different blurred effect.

**Cyclists,
Siem Riep, Cambodia**

Groups of cyclists passed by this area every evening around sunset. I waited at the spot for an hour, shooting a number of frames until I believed I had a strong combination of people, light and movement.

◀ 35mm SLR, 85mm lens, 1/8 f16, Ektachrome E100G

Motion with Flash

Flash can make panning and blurring even more dynamic. It's best to shoot with a slow shutter speed, perhaps 1/15 of a second or slower. The flash freezes the motion of a person in mid-action but there is movement and blur everywhere else.

Wedding, Singapore

Flash and a slow shutter speed capture a sense of movement as the wedding procession passes through the temple. I panned the camera at the same speed as the procession to avoid too much movement.

▲ DSLR, 17-35mm lens at 35mm, 1/10 f3.5, 200 ISO, 2240 x 1488, JPEG

DETAILS

A detail of an individual can show more than the whole and stir the imagination. It's not always essential to photograph people with a full-length or three-quarter-length framing or in a close-up facial portrait. Rather, a good photograph can be achieved by capturing an all-important detail. Laughing eyes, prayer beads in a hand, ribbons in hair, body tattoos or dancing feet are only some of the ways to express everything you wish to say about the essence, mood or spirit of a person.

Window light, side light and back light all work well for revealing close-up details and textures of the human body. A detail, a part of the whole, is a wonderful way of capturing a unique image of a person.

Sheriff's midriff, USA

I saw this sheriff leaning against a wall and talking to his friends. I asked him about his ornate belt and he asked me if I would like to photograph it.

◀ 35mm SLR, 24mm lens, Ektachrome E100SW

Hands with rose, Singapore

It's not always necessary to take an overall picture of the event. Sometimes a close-up or detail can say enough.

▼ DSLR, 17-35mm lens at 35mm, 1/400 f5, 400 ISO, 2240 x 1488, JPEG

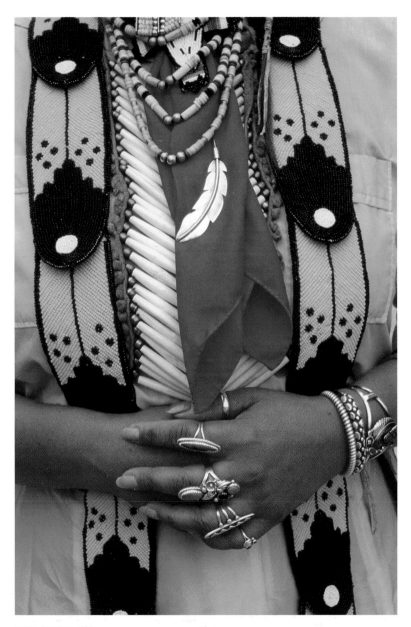

Native American, USA

In this picture I focussed on the woman's silver jewellery. Anything more or less would have ruined the composition.

▲ 35mm SLR, 35mm lens, Ektachrome E100SW

HUMOUR

Always remember to keep your sense of humour when photographing people. You're far more likely to capture quirky, whimsical and funny images if you enjoy what you're doing. Humour itself is difficult to define. Look for unlikely or improbable juxtapositions of subject, background, intent or circumstance that in combination are humorous. For example, pictures of people sleeping when they should be awake or alert, or a person walking past a large poster and wearing something in contrast to what is behind them. In general, humorous pictures tend to be spontaneous and therefore a bonus in your collection of travel photos. However, be on the lookout for a situation or circumstance that might lend itself to the humorous or the absurd, and wait and watch.

Man kissing camel, Darwin, Australia

My assignment was to photograph this camel breeder with his animals. When he walked up to the camels they were so pleased to see him that they leaned over and kissed him. When travelling, always be ready with your camera because you never know what's going to happen.

▲ 35mm SLR, 24mm lens, 1/125 f5.6, Kodachrome 64

Sleeping in rickshaw, Melaka, Malaysia

This man was resting in his rickshaw during the heat of the midday sun. His mouth was open and he was snoring, oblivious to the tourists passing by.

◄ DSLR, 17-35mm lens at 24mm, 1/100 f3.5, 200 ISO, 3008 x 2000, RAW

FURTHER READING

Many of the books that influenced the author are no longer in print, but they may be purchased second-hand from www.amazon.com or www.ebay.com.

Burian, Peter K,
and Robert Caputo
National Geographic Photography
Field Guide
National Geographic, 2003

Busselle, Michael
Better Picture Guide to Photographing
People
Rotovision, 1999

Calder, Julian,
and John Garrett
The New 35mm Photographer's
Handbook
Three Rivers Press, 1999

Caputo, Robert
National Geographic Photography
Field Guide: People & Portraits
National Geographic, 2002

Curtin, Dennis P,
and Steve Musselman
Into Your Darkroom Step By Step
Amherst Media, 1991

Freeman, John
The Photographer's Guide to
Portraits
Collins & Brown, 2004

Freeman, John
Photography
Collins & Brown, 2003

Freeman, Michael
Photographing People
Ilex, 2003

Garrett, John
Black and White Photography
Masterclass
Collins & Brown, 2000

Hedgecoe, John
Photographing People
Collins & Brown, 2000

Hedgecoe, John
Portraits
Collins & Brown, 2000

I'Anson, Richard
Travel Photography:
A Guide to Taking Better Pictures
Lonely Planet Publications, 2004

Krist, Bob
Spirit of Place:
The Art of the Traveling Photographer
Amphoto, 2000

Langford, Michael
35mm Handbook
Knopf, 1993

Lista, Duren,
and Will McDonald
Build Your Own Home Darkroom
Amherst Media, 1990

USEFUL WEBSITES

AgfaPhoto
http://agfaphoto.com

Canon
http://canon.com

Rob Galbraith Digital Insights
www.robgalbraith.com

Eastman Kodak
http://kodak.com

Fujifilm Worldwide
http://home.fujifilm.com

Ilford
www.ilford.com

Lonely Planet
www.lonelyplanet.com

Konica Minolta
http://minolta.com

National Geographic Society
http://nationalgeographic.com

Nevada Wier
www.nevadawier.com

Nikon
http://nikon.com

Olympus
http://olympus.com

Pentax
http://pentax.com

Dan Heller Photography
www.danheller.com

PhotoSecrets
http://photosecrets.com

Travel-Library.com
http://travel-library.com

Tamrac
www.tamrac.com

INDEX

bold refers to image captions

NOTES

NOTES

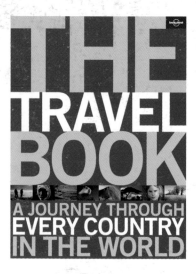

The Travel Book

1 74104 451 0
265mm x 355mm   US$39.99 | UK£40.00

The definitive pictorial dedicated to travel and the world, *The Travel Book* captures every country on the planet in stunning photographs and atmospheric text. Inspirational, inviting and beautiful, it includes user-friendly A-to-Z coverage, with double-page spreads, of every country in the world.

One Planet (hardback)

1 74104 452 9
200mm x 200mm   US$19.99 | UK£14.99

Awesome landscapes, intimate rituals, extreme adventures and moments of connection – *One Planet* is a celebration of life, curiosity and the experience of travel.

This gift hardback edition of Lonely Planet's best-selling pictorial, *One Planet* (September 2003), inspires the reader to explore their passion for travel.

One Planet Postcards

1 74104 453 7
170mm x 120mm   US$11.99 | UK£7.99

A book of 30 compelling postcards handpicked from Lonely Planet's best-selling pictorial *One Planet* (September 2003), celebrating the release of the 2004 gift hardback edition. This book of postcards underscores the importance of connection by inspiring written communication between friends and fellow travellers.

Rice Trails

1 74104 309 3
240mm x 300mm   US$40.00 | UK£25.00

2004 is the 'International Year of Rice' – UN Food & Agriculture Organization

Rice is the world's most important food but also the most fundamental. This hardcover is a beautifully conceived pictorial dedicated to everything to do with this vital food source.